THE CBD HANDBOOK

THE CBD HANDBOOK

Karin Mallion BSc (Hons) MNIMH

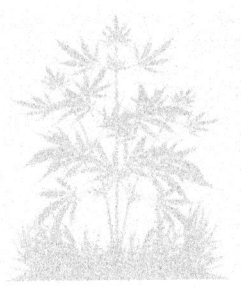

AEON

First published in 2021 by
Aeon Books
Hilltop
Lewes BN7 3HS

Copyright © 2021 by Karin Mallion

The right of Karin Mallion to be identified as the author of this work has been asserted in accordance with §§ 77 and 78 of the Copyright Design and Patents Act 1988.

All rights reserved. No part of this publication may be reproduced, stored in a retrieval system, or transmitted, in any form or by any means, electronic, mechanical, photocopying, recording, or otherwise, without the prior written permission of the publisher.

British Library Cataloguing in Publication Data

A C.I.P. for this book is available from the British Library

ISBN-13: 978-1-91280-761-1

Typeset by Medlar Publishing Solutions Pvt Ltd, India
Printed in Great Britain

www.aeonbooks.co.uk

*The healing comes from nature and
not from the physician, therefore the
physician must start from nature,
with an open mind ...*
~ *Paracelsus*

*It has been quite a journey writing this book,
through some very turbulent times and
I have had help from some amazing friends
and family members. I would like to thank
Emma Dalton for always being there with
wisdom and inspiration and keeping me going!
Thanks also to Bev Harrow, for your inimitable
sense of humour, your encyclopaedic
knowledge, and your friendship.*

CONTENTS

INTRODUCTION xiii

Chapter 1

What is CBD? (history and overview) 1
    Prior to Christianity 2
    Post-Christianity..4
    Recent history—nineteenth and twentieth centuries............5
    Western medical use of cannabis in the
        twentieth century 9
    Modern thinking 10

Chapter 2

What can CBD help with?.. 13

Chapter 3

Cannabinoids..17
    What are cannabinoids? 17
    What is THC? (tetrahydracannabinol).................................18
    What is CBD (cannabidiol)? 20
    What is anandamide? 22
    The role of anandamide 24

Pain relief..24
Reward..24
The "runner's high"..24
Mood enhancement..25
Reproduction and fertility...............................25
Breast milk..26
Cell regulation and development....................26
Is it possible to increase anandamide?.....................27
What is CBN? (cannabinol)...27
What is CBG? (cannabigerol).....................................28
What is CBDV? (cannabidivarin)...............................30
What is CBC? (cannabichromene).............................31
What is THCV? (tetrahydrocannabivarin)................33

Chapter 4

The endocannabinoid system...35
Balancing the endocannabinoid system..................39
Stress response...39
Dietary response..40
Drugs and alcohol..41
Genetic predisposition.......................................41
Restoring the balance..41
Phytocannabinoids...42
CBD and its interaction with the
endocannabinoid system...................................42
The biphasic effect...43
The Herxheimer reaction..................................44

Chapter 5 47

The CB-1 and CB-2 receptors..47
What are CB-1 receptors?...47
What are CB-2 receptors?...49

Chapter 6

Metabolism 51
   The endocannabinoid system and homeostasis 51
   Metabolisation and CYP450 interaction 53
      THC metabolisation 55
      What does this mean for herb–drug
      interactions? 55

Chapter 7

Indica or sativa—what is the difference? 57
   The anticipated effects of an "indica" or "sativa"
      strain of plant 60
      Indica chemovar subtype 61
      Sativa chemovar subtype 62
      Hybrid chemovars 62

Chapter 8

Plant secondary metabolites—terpenes/terpenoids 65
   Common terpenes found in cannabis plants 66
   Individual terpenes—a closer look 69
      Myrcene 69
   Linalool 70
   Limonene 72
   Caryophyllene 73
   Pinene 75
      So how does pinene work? 76
   Humulene 77
   Terpinolene 78
   Camphene 79
   Phellandrene 80
   Carene 81

Terpineol..82
Pulegone..82
Sabinene...83
Geraniol..84

Chapter 9

Flavonoids and cannaflavins... 85
    The many health benefits of flavonoids............................87
    Flavonoids and cancer...88
    Flavonoids and cannabis..90
    The "entourage effect" 91

Chapter 10

Herbs that work synergistically with cannabis 93
        Cannabis and lavender..94
        Cannabis and rosemary...94
        Cannabis and holy basil..95
        Cannabis and echinacea...96
        Cannabis and black cohosh 96
        Cannabis and ashwagandha..97
        Synergy between ashwagandha and CBD 98
        Cannabis and turmeric..99
        Cannabis and cacao 100

Chapter 11

Cannabis and cancer—The Cancer Act of 1939 103

Chapter 12

Studies on the effects of CBD in pets.......................................105

Chapter 13

What to look for when purchasing CBD?...............................109

Chapter 14

Delivery methods and contraindications 115
    Inhalation 115
    Oral ingestion 117
    Sublingual 118
    Topical application... 118
    How to take CBD oil.. 120
    CBD interactions with other herbs
        or pharmaceuticals.. 121
    Antibiotics... 122
    Chemotherapy.. 123
    Antidepressants and anti-anxiety medicines................... 123
    Blood thinners 123
    Ibuprofen.. 124
    Topical CBD 124

Chapter 15

Health conditions and their responses to CBD..................... 125
    Priming the endocannabinoid system 126
    Conditions.. 126
    Pain relief.. 128
    Attention deficit disorder and attention deficit
        hyperactivity disorder... 129
    Anxiety, stress, and depression.. 130
    Arthritis 133
    Rheumatoid arthritis 133
    Behçet's disease 135
    Collagen connective tissue disorders.............................. 136
    COPD.. 138
    Epilepsy 140

Fibromyalgia and polymyalgia rheumatica 141
PCOS 142
PMDD/PMS 143
Irritable bowel, ulcerative colitis, and other
    gastrointestinal conditions 144
Menopause 145
Migraines 147
Multiple sclerosis 148
Skin conditions 150
Sleep 150
Spinal cord injury 150
Sciatica and piriformis syndrome 152

Chapter 16

CBD as a daily general health supplement 153
CBD for athletes 153
Is it possible for a professional athlete to use CBD? 154
    Information regarding COVID-19—the
        coronavirus 155
    Long COVID 157

Chapter 17

CBD in practice—a few testimonials and stories 159
Fibromyalgia and cancer—testimonial 160
Anxiety and post cancer malaise 164
Severe mental health concerns 165
Chronic regional pain syndrome—testimonial 166
    Fast forward 12 months 167
    Polypharmacy and pain 168

BIBLIOGRAPHY 169

INDEX 185

INTRODUCTION

CBD is the "buzz word" product in the UK with an estimated 1000 new users each month. Press reports have abounded regarding the efficacy of CBD and its "wonder drug" healing properties for almost any ailment, from cancer through to epilepsy, multiple sclerosis to headaches, anxiety, and probably hangnails! CBD is shorthand for canabidiol, an active but not intoxicating ingredient of medical marijuana (cannabis).

The number of people using this substance is ever growing, but there seems to be a great deal of confusion about what it actually does, how to use it, herb–prescription drug interactions, and the difference between different products. Our television screens and newspapers have been deluged with a profusion of vastly differing stories and it has featured on various consumer programmes such as *Trust Me, I'm a Doctor* and the investigation of the *Gogglebox* "couple" (Steph and Dom Parker), who wanted to use CBD to help their son with epilepsy. There was even a programme where a group of celebrities drove around the United States in a flower-power bus sampling a variety of different substances, visiting cannabis pharmacies and growers. These media reports have increased the public's appetite for CBD exponentially.

However, there is still such a great lack of knowledge, information, and guidance about this product in the UK, with an abundance of "internet help forums" springing up and many manufacturers of "CBD oil" products trying to get onto the bandwagon—often with products of dubious quality and vague ingredients. Many manufacturers are using "isolates"—that is, making use of an extracted CBD and not whole plant extract: these contain no other cannabinoids and are far cheaper to buy than the superior whole plant extract products. However, it gives many small companies a chance to get into what they perceive as the lucrative CBD market without a large investment.

As a medical herbalist, I am, of course, interested in CBD and cannabis, although my personal use had been distinctly limited—the usual late teenage attempts, which always resulted in significant malaise: the wobbliness, nausea, and a general "seasick feeling" that cannabis gave me meant it was not for me. But in 2017 everyone was talking about it, and as a health shop owner, manufacturers were contacting me with their various products to try with my clients and patients. I became more interested and began to stock some of these products, noting that some had better effects on some patients than on others. The descriptions on the containers were all different; there seemed to be no uniformity across the products. However, I did notice that some products produced little to no effect while some had a significant effect. My first "amazing" result was with a customer who had been diagnosed with prostate cancer and whose prostate-specific antigen markers were extremely high. Within three months of using an over the counter product from my little health shop, his PSA markers were in the normal range and the cancer was operable and he made a complete recovery. Both the customer and I were stunned that a few drops of oil could have this marked effect.

At that time, I was not just running my own health shop but also working part-time for an herbal medicine supplier and manufacturer. I had been discussing the results I was seeing through CBD products with my colleagues, and between us we decided it was time to offer this product to medical herbalists so that they could buy it from the same place they buy their herbal supplies—as a "one-stop shop".

An enormous selection and variety of CBD products is now available in the UK marketplace, some from dubious and some from not so dubious sources. There are slanderous allegations, power struggles, and spiteful infighting within these various companies. I have seen everything from CBD chewing gum and drinks, to lotions, potions, capsules, massage oils, and sublingual oils, and many more. There are even CBD pillows touted to give you a better night's sleep! Herbalists have been using hops and lavender in sachets and pillows for years, but they don't appear to have quite the pizazz that accompanies CBD.

Meanwhile, back in 2017, I had contacted several manufacturers of CBD oil products and asked if I could visit them, and perhaps see how they made their product and learn more about it. What was worrying to me was that there were so very many different products available—and my patients did not know which one was the best. Very importantly no one was able to give them information regarding contraindications with existing medication, or even what this product could do for them. The manufacturers have their hands tied as under the terms of the Medicine and Health Regulatory Authority they are not able to say "what the product is good for" and it is only sold as a "food supplement" or "health supplement"—because of the sensitive nature of it being "cannabis" the government has been cautious with its regulations. These companies are suppliers and manufacturers, not medical professionals, and thus cannot give medical advice.

Equally, medical herbalists and homeopaths, osteopaths and acupuncturists, and other complementary practitioners are not trained in the benefits or contraindications of cannabis when used in this way. The herbal manufacturer I was working with thought it would be a good idea to research more about the product and put together a presentation for herbalists that would give them an indication of what could be supported or helped using cannabis extracts.

As my interest in cannabis and CBD grew, and I saw the results that both my family and patients were seeing from the use of cannabis, at the behest of my employers, Planta Medica Ltd, I wrote a seminar contribution to discuss the therapeutic implications of cannabis, which I presented in the spring of 2018 to a group of medical herbalists. This talk became so popular that my colleague Emma Dalton and I ended up presenting to a variety of herbalists, homeopaths, kinesiologists, GPs, nurses, and other medical and complementary practitioners. These were extremely well attended and demand and bookings for these talks flowed in.

I was subsequently offered employment by one of the CBD companies with an opportunity to go to the island of Guernsey to set up a herbal practice and a shop with herbal remedies, selling a range of high-quality cannabis extracts to the general public. Because of the previously mentioned legislation and rules set by the MHRA and the fact that manufacturers were unable to say anything about their products and could make no medicinal claims, the issue was how should the manufacturers advise their customers which product to use, and how might it help them with various health concerns? This is confusing for therapists and consumers alike. It was considered that my status as a medical herbalist put me in a good position to advise people as to which products to use and how to use them.

I stayed in Guernsey for around fifteen months—a wonderful experience seeing thousands of patients and customers, many of whom became regulars, so it was possible to see improvements in health and hear their stories and experiences. I returned to England in the autumn of 2019 and continued to work with Planta Medica who by this point had bought extraction machinery, set up laboratories, and were looking at manufacturing a product from scratch—so that the herbalists who bought its products would be assured of high quality and purity without the doubt that attaches to some of the other companies selling these products. We launched the company Cannamedica in January 2020 (just before the first COVID-19 lockdown was imposed).

What follows is mostly a compilation of literature collated from books, a wide variety of internet sites, personal experience, and case histories. I hope you find it useful.

Karin Mallion BSc (Hons) MNIMH, medical herbalist
November 2020

CHAPTER 1

What is CBD?
(history and overview)

Cannabidiol (CBD) is one of over 100 cannabinoids found in cannabis, but it is the one that has been found to be particularly beneficial to well-being and without many negative health side effects. Most CBD products are grown from cannabis/hemp and the extract or oil is used as a food supplement to help improve and maintain health.

Historically hemp was an agricultural crop, utilised mostly in Europe for its fibres such as in making rope and fishing

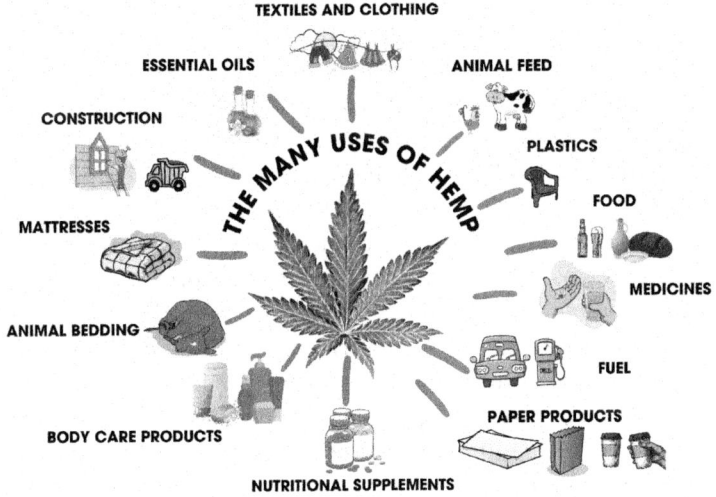

nets, and for weaving into strong hardwearing textiles. Before cotton, it was used to make clothes, sails, and other fabric products. Hemp requires fewer chemicals and less processing than cotton to make it useable. Its seed can be eaten whole, ground into flour, or pressed to produce a highly nutritious oil. A hundred years ago, hemp was one of the most commonly grown agricultural crops. It was part of our daily diet as well as being used for its fibre and medicinal purposes. The leaves can be used as any other green vegetable and its flowers contain powerful compounds used as medicine to treat all sorts of ailments. In the late 1900s, more than half of all pharmacy medicines contained cannabis.

Prior to Christianity

Cannabis sativa (cannabis) is one of the earliest cultivated plants. Evidence indicates cannabis was first found in China. Archaeologists have discovered that the plant was grown and used for its fibres from around 4000 BC. The Chinese used it for manufacturing rope, textiles, and paper, and evidence of this was found in the tomb of Emperor Wu (106–87 BC), dating back to the Han dynasty.

The fruits of the cannabis plant were also used in Chinese culture as a food ingredient, although the food use of cannabis had declined by the beginning of the Christian era. Using cannabis as a medicine by the Ancient Chinese is recorded in the *Pen-Ts'ao Ching*, an ancient pharmacopoeia which was based on oral traditions passed down from around 2700 BC. Cannabis was used as a medicine to treat rheumatic pain, constipation, female reproductive disorders, malaria, and more. The founder of Chinese surgery, Hua T'o (110–207 AD), used a compound mixture including cannabis (to be taken with wine) to anaesthetise his patients during surgery. Predominantly the Chinese used hemp seeds for medicinal purposes, especially as a laxative and for skin conditions. The seeds are devoid in tetrahydrocannabinol (THC), the main psychoactive compound in cannabis; however, they do have important properties containing essential fatty acids such as g-linoleic acid (omega 6).

Early references to cannabis being used as a psychoactive drug are also to be found in the *Pen-Ts'ao Ching* ("The Divine Farmer's Materia Medica"), "Ma-fen [fruits of hemp] … if taken in excess will produce hallucinations [literally, seeing devils]." On the other hand, moderate use over a longer time has benefits. "taken over the long term, it makes one communicate with spirits and lightens one's body." This is a rare reference to cannabis in this form from this historical period, and particularly rare in the Ancient Chinese pharmacopoeia. It is thought that this may be because the use of cannabis as a psychoactive drug was restricted to shamanism which was declining in China but far more common in the northern nomadic tribes, western Asia, and in India.

Cannabis was widely used in India. An ancient Hindu scripture, the *Atharva Veda*, names cannabis as a sacred plant; a bringer of freedom, happiness, and joy, and thus cannabis became ensconced within religious rituals and was widely used as both a medicine and a recreational drug. In India, there were reputed to be at least three different preparations of the plant: *Bhang* which consisted of only dried leaves, from which flowers were removed; *Ganja* made only from the flowers; and an extremely strong variation called *Charas* which was made only from the resin that covers the female flowers. It is considered likely that medicinal and religious use of cannabis dates back to around 1000 BC and had a wide variety of uses and applications including as an analgesic, anti-convulsant, hypnotic, tranquilliser, anaesthetic, anti-inflammatory, antiparasitic, antispasmodic, antitussive, expectorant, and antibiotic.

There are historical references inferring that cannabis was considered sacred and utilised in Tibet, especially to facilitate meditation. The Tibetan medicine was based upon Hindu medicine and botany was considered particularly important—it is reported that cannabis grew prolifically in that region. The Ancient Assyrians were also purported to have used cannabis probably from around the ninth century BC, with early evidence indicating that prior to the Christian era cannabis was used both externally for bruising or swellings and internally for a variety of conditions including depression and arthritis.

Early Persians knew of the plant prior to the Christian era, whilst in Europe archaeological evidence suggests that cannabis was used in some form. Charred cannabis seeds were found in Scythian tombs in Siberia and Germany and it is mooted that these were used during funeral ceremonies to be inhaled for ritualistic purposes. There is, however, scant evidence to suggest use of the plant by either the Greeks or Romans.

There is significant evidence to show the use of cannabis in Ancient Egypt, with depictions of the goddess Seshat (Goddess of Wisdom) showing a cannabis leaf above her head. Mummies such as the Pharaoh Rameses II and many others were found with traces of cannabis in the remains. The Ebers Papyrus from the National Library of Medicine found in Egypt in the 1870s showed a prescription for an asthma remedy which involved the preparation of various herbs, including cannabis to be heated on a brick so that the sufferer could inhale the fumes.

Post-Christianity

Cannabis continued to be used prolifically in India, spreading gradually to the Middle East and Africa. The well-known Persian polymath and physician Ibn Sina (Avicenna) mentioned the use of cannabis in his medical texts around the year 1000 AD. Its properties were considered to be diuretic, digestive, and "to clean the brain" as well as soothing earache. The Arab world initially embraced the use of cannabis, with one writer, Ibn Bukhari, saying in the eleventh century that the juice from cannabis leaves could cure an abscess in the head; a century later another (Ibn-al-Baytar) suggested that the oil from cannabis seeds could remove hardened tumours. However, by the beginning of the thirteenth century, the Arab world banned the use of cannabis based upon the teachings of Islam; even so, there are reports from Ibn al-Badri in 1464 claiming that the epileptic son of the caliph's chamberlain was treated with the resin from the plant and cured completely of his affliction. He, however, further referenced that this made the son "an addict who could not for a moment be without the drug". Historically there are many references citing cannabis as a medicinal aid, for such conditions as amenorrhoea, headaches, haemorrhoids, nerve pain, inflammation, epilepsy, and more.

The use of cannabis as a medicine in Africa has been documented since at least the fifteenth century, potentially introduced by Arabs or Indian traders. Records indicate that it was used to facilitate childbirth, malaria, fever, asthma, and dysentery.

Research shows that they had cannabis seeds in Brazil as early as the sixteenth century, brought over by African slaves, and reports cite its use in religious rituals and for toothache and menstrual cramps. Meanwhile in Europe the plant was mainly cultivated for its fibres for use in the making of cloth, sails, rope, and paper.

Although the ancient Egyptians used papyrus upon which to write, the early Chinese invented "paper" made from hemp and wood pulp, which they then introduced to India and the Arab world who then later introduced it to Europe.

Recent history—nineteenth and twentieth centuries

In the early nineteenth century, there is some reference to the use of cannabis medicinally, but in the middle of the century an Irish physician by the name of William O'Shaughnessy discovered cannabis while serving in India with the British Army. After some years of study, evaluation, and testing on patients with various pathologies, he published a work entitled "On the preparations of the Indian hemp, or gunjah". O'Shaughnessy expounded the use of hemp in various forms for a variety of conditions listing rheumatism, convulsions, and muscular spasms as well as rabies and tetanus.

At around the same time a French psychiatrist named Jacques-Joseph Moreau who through his work for the Charenton Asylum near Paris travelled extensively to exotic countries with his patients. It was through this work that he discovered the use of cannabis resin (hashish) which was in common use in the Orient. He was surprised at the effects of the plant and experimented prolifically on himself and patients, later writing a book about the effects of cannabis upon mental disorders and its alleviation of many symptoms and comorbidities. The works of these two men were hugely important in the nineteenth century and by 1860 the first clinical conference about cannabis took place, organised by the Ohio State Medical Society in America.

DU HACHISCH

ET DE

L'ALIÉNATION MENTALE

ÉTUDES PSYCHOLOGIQUES

PAR

J. MOREAU
(DE TOURS),
Médecin de l'hospice de Bicêtre, Membre de la Société
orientale de Paris.

PARIS.
LIBRAIRIE DE FORTIN, MASSON ET C⁽ⁱᵉ⁾.
PLACE DE L'ÉCOLE-DE-MÉDECINE, 1,
Même maison, chez Léopold Michelsen, à Leipzig.

1845.

Influenced by William O'Shaughnessy, legend has it that Queen Victoria's own physician, Sir John Russell Reynolds prescribed cannabis for the Queen to help with menstrual pains, although there are few references to support this, other than Reynolds's own articles in *The Lancet* stating that "cannabis when pure and administered carefully, is one of the most valuable medicines we possess". This "fact" is used frequently in documentation supporting the historical use of cannabis, although sadly, some deeper research has uncovered the point that by the time Reynolds became physician to the Royal Household, Victoria would have been sixty, and therefore unlikely to suffer menstrual pains. That is not to say that one of her previous doctors did not prescribe it for her as it is known that opium and coca and chloroform were in common use in Victorian times. This particular historical titbit is so popular that it is cited even in academic papers; however, I can find nothing convincingly accurate that fully substantiates it.

By the latter half of the nineteenth century over 100 scientific articles had been published regarding the therapeutic value of cannabis; it was included in tinctures and extracts, and began to be marketed by laboratories such as Merck (Germany), Burroughs-Wellcome (England), and Bristol-Meyers Squibb (United States), amongst others.

At around this same time, vilification of cannabis as a medicine had already begun; the House of Commons in England heard from a Member of Parliament stating, "The lunatic asylums of India are filled with ganja smokers." The House of Commons commissioned a report, and the Government of India created a seven-member group to examine the questions. The Indian Hemp Drugs Commission was formed and produced a very comprehensive report of around 3280 pages around 1894/5, which held testimony from over 1200 "doctors, coolies, yogis, fakirs, heads of lunatic asylums, bhang peasants, tax gatherers, smugglers, army officers, hemp dealers, ganja palace operators and the clergy. The report was considered very thorough and an excerpt states that "It has been clearly established that the occasional use of hemp in moderate doses may be beneficial, but this use may be regarded as medicinal in character." The report further stated that

> In regard to the physical effects, the Commission have come to the conclusion that the moderate use of hemp drugs is practically attended by no evil results at all. There may be exceptional cases in which, owing to idiosyncrasies of constitution, the drugs in even moderate use may be injurious. There is probably nothing the use of which may not possibly be injurious in cases of exceptional intolerance. There are also many cases where in tracts with a specially malarious climate, or in circumstances of hard work and exposure, the people attribute beneficial effects to the habitual moderate use of these drugs; and there is evidence to show that the popular impression may have some basis in fact. Speaking generally, the Commission are of opinion that the moderate use of hemp drugs appears to cause no appreciable physical injury of any kind. The excessive use does cause injury. As in the case of other intoxicants, excessive use tends to weaken the constitution and to render the consumer more susceptible to disease.

In respect of the mental effects of cannabis, the Commission

> have come to the conclusion that the moderate use of hemp drugs produces no injurious effects on the mind. It may indeed be accepted that in the case of specially marked neurotic diathesis, even the moderate use may produce mental injury. For the slightest mental stimulation or excitement may have that effect in such cases. But putting aside these quite exceptional cases, the moderate use of these drugs produces no mental injury.

REPORT

OF THE

INDIAN HEMP DRUGS COMMISSION,

1893-94.

President:

The Hon'ble W. MACKWORTH YOUNG, M.A., C.S.I., First Financial Commissioner, Punjab.

Members:

1. Mr. H. T. OMMANNEY, Collector, Panch Mahals, Bombay.
2. Mr. A. H. L. FRASER, M.A., Commissioner, Chhattisgarh Division, Central Provinces.
3. Surgeon-Major C. J. H. WARDEN, Professor of Chemistry, Medical College, and Chemical Examiner to Government, Calcutta; Officiating Medical Storekeeper to Government, Calcutta.
4. Raja SOSHI SIKHARESWAR ROY, of Tahirpur, Bengal.
5. KANWAR HARNAM SINGH, Ahluwalia, C.I.E., Punjab.
6. LALA NIHAL CHAND, of Muzaffarnagar, North-Western Provinces.

Secretary:

Mr. H. J. McINTOSH, Under-Secretary to the Government of Bengal, Financial and Municipal Departments.

Despite this rather positive view of the medicinal attributes of hemp, the vilification and concern raised by the House of Commons and reported in the press of the day, precipitated the decline of cannabis, the use of which significantly decreased in the early twentieth century.

Western medical use of cannabis in the twentieth century

There was a decline in the medicinal use of cannabis from the beginning of the twentieth century, partly owing to the difficulty of obtaining replicable effects. These varied dramatically depending upon the type of plant, its provenance, and the extraction methods used; whether its seeds

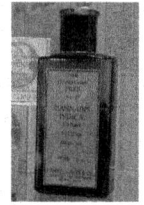

had been dissolved in wine, vinegar, or water; or a tincture created from resin, leaf, or flower. Additionally, the arrival of various other medications, such as aspirin for analgesia, and hypodermic syringes, which allowed the injection of morphine, along with the discovery of barbiturates and substances such as chloral hydrate and paraldehyde, and the discovery of a vaccination for tetanus, for which hemp was often used, meant that cannabis became less popular. Legal restrictions began to limit the use of cannabis, with the "Marijuana Tax Act", a law passed in 1937 in the USA, which required anyone using this plant to register and pay a tax of $1 per ounce if used for medical purposes and $100 per ounce for any other use. Non-payment of the tax resulted in a $2000 fine and/or five years' imprisonment. Owing to the excessive paperwork involved and the punitive measures imposed, use of the plant diminished until it was removed from the *American Pharmacopeia* in 1941.

Socio-economically, however, cannabis use for hedonistic purposes then exploded, where previously it had only been used by a small group of intellectuals and authors in Europe, and by small groups of people in Brazil and in Mexico where it was used by the most underprivileged population. Through the Mexican immigrants, its use for recreational purposes reached the US, and until the 1950s this use was limited to black or Hispanic immigrants. However, its use spread to the young and in the liberated 1960s it became hugely popular: studies show that the percentage of young adults using cannabis rose from around 5% in the early 1960s to over 68% by the end of the decade and its use for recreational purposes remains high to date.

Modern thinking

The Israeli scientist Raphael Mechoulam and his colleague Yehiel Gaoni first isolated THC (tetrahydrocannabinol) from cannabis in 1965, which marks the beginning of a prolific period of studies into cannabinoids and their isolation. For the next five to eight years, scientific interest grew, peaking in the early 1970s. A Brazilian research group led by Dr Elisaldo Carlini researched the interactions of Delta-9 tetrahydrocannabinol, contributing valuable work. Interest in researching cannabis waned in the mid-1970s, but gained momentum again in the early 1990s when Mechoulam isolated anandamide, a cannabinoid produced by the human body, known as an endogenous cannabinoid, and thereby discovered the endocannabinoid system, a series of receptors found in the nervous system and brain.

Scientific interest once more grew, the therapeutic effects of cannabis now being studied with more advanced scientific methods. Studies are ongoing on the therapeutic effects of cannabis, CBD, and THC regarding a variety of conditions including epilepsy, insomnia, multiple sclerosis, Tourette's syndrome, nausea, chemotherapy support, glaucoma, and many more. There is growing evidence that cannabidiol (CBD) can have positive effects upon epilepsy, anxiety, inflammation, psychoses, and neuroprotection. There are, however, studies that suggest that the use of cannabis containing a high level of THC can induce cognitive deficits and create a risk for psychosis among vulnerable young people.

In the mid-2000s a British company, GW Pharmaceuticals, received approval to commence marketing its Sativex product containing a blend of Delta-9 THC and CBD for the relief of neuropathic pain in patients with multiple sclerosis, and most recently it has developed Epidiolex for those suffering from epilepsy.

Some scientists have mooted that because we no longer regularly consume the same quantities of nutritious cannabinoids, terpenes, and flavonoids as our ancestors, this has led to a pandemic of "endocannabinoid system deficiency". Our receptors still recognise the small amounts that can be found in breast milk, broccoli, and echinacea but cannabis is the richest source.

It has been posited that the upsurge in autoimmune conditions, multiple sclerosis, and Crohn's disease could be a result of endocannabinoid deficiency. Which is why a significant amount of research is taking place into using cannabis and cannabinoids to treat these conditions.

Research into the medicinal properties of cannabis is still in its infancy—funding issues, narcotic associations, and public perception continue to hamper quality research, so there are still not enough so-called "evidence-based" papers to be clear as to what exactly cannabis can treat.

Hemp must be legally grown under licence and selectively bred to produce low levels of THC. In the UK industrial hemp must contain less than 0.2% THC; in the US the limit is 0.3%. However, in October 2020, the European Parliament voted to increase the level of THC permitted in legal industrial hemp from 0.2 to 0.3 per cent. Whether this will be adopted by the UK is still unclear (at time of writing). A great deal of CBD oil is produced from the lower leaves and not the flowers or buds which would not be defined as industrial hemp by UK law.

However, it still contains all the important ingredients which are highly nutritious and healthy such as cannabidiol (CBD) and other cannabinoids, terpenes, and flavonoids.

Cannabidiol (CBD) oil is not the same as hempseed oil and it is particularly important to understand the difference.

Hempseed oil is made by pressing the seeds and is a highly nutritious but delicate oil containing a balance of omega 3 and 6 which is almost perfect for human consumption, but it contains only trace amounts of cannabinoids. It is great for salad dressings, baking, and low-temperature cooking but not for frying or cooking at high temperatures. For the same reason it is not a good oil for use as a fuel or biodiesel.

CHAPTER 2

What can CBD help with?

No company in the UK should be promoting CBD for medicinal use—as the MHRA have designated that if it has a medicinal use then it should only be prescribed by a doctor. However, CBD is one of the fastest-selling supplements in both the US and the UK. CBD is non-polar (i.e. it is not water soluble and it requires alcohol or another substance for extraction) and in the UK it is usually mixed with olive oil, hemp oil, or fractionated coconut/MCT for dilution. For those of us who are medical herbalists, a tincture would be a substance extracted in ethanol; however, extracted CBD oil is also called a tincture by the manufacturers, which I initially found very confusing.

Most manufacturers will not list a string of ailments that "CBD can help with" as this goes against the advice of the Home Office and Medicine and Health Regulatory Authority; however, soon after the ITV showing of a programme called "Gone to Pot", I received an email from an online supplement supplier which listed the benefits of taking CBD as follows.

Joint pain:

CBD hemp extracts are antioxidant and have anti-inflammatory effects on joints, to help improve pain and stiffness. They also have pain-relieving effects due to their interaction with certain parts of the brain.

Anxiety:

Cannabidiol helps to reduce muscle tension, restlessness and fatigue. In a study involving people with social anxiety, taking CBD supplements before a public speaking engagement reduced anxiety, muddled thoughts, social discomfort, and anticipatory anxiety significantly more than a placebo. CBD may also help with the anxiety that can occur when stopping smoking.

Panic attacks:

Cannabidiol is being investigated as a promising treatment for panic attacks, obsessive compulsive disorder and post-traumatic stress disorder.

Sleep:

Cannabidiol (CBD) is a popular treatment for insomnia and promotes refreshing REM sleep and reduced excessive daytime sleepiness. REM sleep means "Rapid Eye Movement" and is essentially the term used for when we enter into a deep phase of sleep—when you dream, you are experiencing REM sleep.

General well-being:

As discussed, CBD oil helps to lift mood and promotes general feelings of well-being.

This list (taken verbatim from the online catalogue of a supplement supplier) despite the statements being illegal, at least gives something to base a customer's decision upon when deciding whether to take CBD oil or not. It is not an exclusive list, and since using CBD oil with patients, I have personally seen many other benefits that are not included in the above description, but it intrigued me enough to want to find out more about cannabis extracts and what they could do for my patients. During my time dealing with patients and customers wanting to try cannabinoid products, they have arrived with a mind-boggling array of ailments that they hope will be magically cured by this much-vaunted substance.

CHAPTER 3

Cannabinoids

What are cannabinoids?

The cannabis plant contains a variety of compounds. I explain it to my patients with my "cake analogy". Trying to explain secondary metabolites to laypeople is simply too technical and scientific for most. So, I explain that "plants are like cakes, they have lots of ingredients, called phytochemicals" (I will come back to this analogy later in Chapter 7). Cannabinoids are compounds found naturally within cannabis plants and each plant contains almost 500 different "ingredients" (phytochemicals). Over 100 of these ingredients are called "cannabinoids".

Within the body, we have an "endocannabinoid system" (there is a chapter about the endocannabinoid system later), but in brief, this endocannabinoid system contains receptors which not only produce the body's own "cannabinoids" but which also react to the cannabinoids we ingest. By facilitating communication between cells endocannabinoids enhance the body's ability to keep itself balanced. Cannabinoids we take exogenously attempt to modulate the compounds our bodies already naturally produce. When these compounds are activated or produced, they can assist in preserving stability within the body and thereby promoting "homeostasis" (balance within the body). As has been posited previously, a deficiency of the "naturally produced" cannabinoids (endocannabinoids) within the system will result in imbalance, and thus create negative symptoms or physical difficulties.

Operating on a kind of lock and key system, on consumption, cannabinoids bind to receptor sites on cells throughout the entire system; these are known as CB-1 (brain) and CB-2 (body) receptors. Depending upon which cannabinoid is ingested, there is a variance in the receptors these bind to. This allows for a certain amount of targeted "medicinal aid" by choosing carefully which product contains the most suitable cannabinoid for the condition. For example, THC binds strongly to receptors in the brain, whereas CBN has more of an affinity with the receptors found throughout the body.

What follows is a list of some of the more well-known cannabinoids.

What is THC? (tetrahydracannabinol)

The discovery of THC is generally ascribed to the Israeli scientist Raphael Mechoulam in the early 1960s. However, there is evidence that THC was used in the 1940s as a kind of truth serum used by the US government and discovered by an American organic chemist named Roger Adams from the University of Illinois. He carried out more than twenty-seven studies on cannabis, published in the *American Journal of Chemistry* between 1940 and 1949. By the 1960s, however, equipment was more advanced and Mechoulam had the advantage of nuclear magnetic resonance spectroscopy and thus was able to further isolate and investigate THC. He is therefore often hailed as the man who discovered THC. THC is one of the most researched, analysed, and effective cannabinoids and it has been attributed with therapeutic value for many different ailments.

- In 1996 a study showed that THC initiates cell apoptosis in tumours and could thereby potentially halt the development of such tumours.
- In 2006, it was revealed (something those who had been using cannabis recreationally already knew) that THC stimulates the appetite which could make it an ideal candidate for use with anorexia, cachexia, and bulimia. Which explains why those who use the drug recreationally are often hungry or have "the munchies" after smoking it.
- Studies have shown that THC blocks pathways through the central nervous system, thereby preventing pain signals through the brain and thus it could be used as a valuable pain-relieving product.
- In the late 1990s it was discovered that the use of THC reduced intraocular pressure in glaucoma patients by up to 65%. But it transpired that these effects were temporary and without continued use would dissipate. Continuous use of high dosage THC could result in toxic systemic effects. Studies continue to try to find a way to prolong the effects without side effects.
- The University of Illinois (alma mater of Roger Adams) has performed some studies which indicate that THC stabilises autonomic output during sleep and thus reduces

spontaneous sleep-disordered breathing. It simultaneously blocks serotonin-induced exacerbation of certain sleep disorders such as sleep apnoea.
- The Virginia Commonwealth University published a study suggesting that the binding of THC onto CB-1 receptors reduces the duration and gravity of seizures in epileptic test subjects.
- A study published in the *Journal of Molecular Pharmaceutics* in 2006 has posited that the enzymes which are key pathological markers in the development of Alzheimer's disease are inhibited by THC.

What is CBD (cannabidiol)?

Cannabis has such a wide variety of different strains that breeders have successfully created many varieties with varying levels of CBD or THC. Some are high in CBD and low in THC; these are mostly the ones that are used for the manufacture of CBD oils.

Cannabidiol has an extremely wide array of medicinal properties and has no psychoactive effects, unlike its relative THC. This lack of psychoactive effects, and the discovery that on its own CBD has therapeutic benefits, have now caused vast popularity and there is hope that this could become a genuine therapeutic.

- Many studies have indicated that CBD has anti-emetic properties—and in fact, a synthetic version, dronabinol, is widely available to combat nausea, sleep apnoea, migraines, vomiting, and also for patients with anorexia nervosa as an appetite stimulant. A Canadian report has indicated that by "manipulating" the endocannabinoid system with CBD the nausea and vomiting in chemotherapy patients can be reduced more effectively than with any other pharmaceutical drug.
- In 2010 a report of a study was published citing antidepressant properties linked to CBD. Tests on animal models revealed that CBD had the same antidepressant effects as imipramine, a popular pharmaceutical antidepressant medicine, without the potentially life-threatening side effects.
- Prolific research on CBD and how it may affect cancer shows that there are potentially anti-cancer and anti-tumour properties to this compound. Using an in-vitro study, scientists found that CBD induced programmed cell apoptosis in breast cancer, completely independent of CB-1 and CB-2 receptors. Other studies have shown, using a mouse model, that CBD could prevent pre-malignant and malignant tumours in the colon and furthermore that it had chemoprotective properties.
- In 2009 a study concluded that CBD had anti-convulsant properties in animal models: "CBD (100 mg/kg) exerted clear anti-convulsant effects with significant decreases in incidence of severe seizures and mortality compared with vehicle-treated [control] animals." It was also found during these trials that CBD worked independently of the CB-1 receptor, which could help infer true legitimacy to CBD in

its ability to be used as an anti-seizure medication for cases of epilepsy. The UK company GW Pharmaceuticals has now developed Epidiolex, an anti-epilepsy alternative, which is awaiting approval and expected to be available on prescription by 2020.

- A news report published by CNN news in the US by a Dr Sanjay Gupta discussed the case of a little girl named Charlotte Figi. Charlotte began having seizures when she was just a few months old and was diagnosed finally with Dravet's syndrome—this took a long time, despite the parents being in Colorado—a state where medical cannabis is available. Her father was in the US Army and very anti-drugs, but the child was suffering severely, and faced likely death, having flatlined in the hospital several times during her extreme seizures. All conventional treatment failed, and some of the pharmaceuticals prescribed to the child had significant side effects; one even caused her to stop breathing. The parents, at their wit's end, decided to use medical cannabis. Charlotte's condition improved dramatically with the oral use of medical CBD rich cannabis, and public interest surged.

What is anandamide?

Anandamide is an "endocannabinoid"—that is to say, it is produced by the body itself.

Anandamide has significant and wide-reaching effects within the body because it interacts with the endocannabinoid system. Its function is to enhance reward, mood, appetite, and pain relief, and it is involved in the reproductive system among many other things.

Anandamide is a neurotransmitter, which binds to CB-1 and CB-2 receptors. It also affects the TRPV-1 (transient receptor potential cation channel subfamily V member 1—also known as the capsaicin receptor or vanilloid receptor 1) which is a genetic protein that detects and regulates body temperature, sensations of scalding heat or pain. Its activation leads to a painful burning sensation and is affected by a variety of endogenous and exogenous stimuli, such as capsaicin, temperatures above 43 degrees Celsius, low PH (acidic) conditions, as well as forms of dopamine. It is modulated by anandamide.

Within the body's endocannabinoid system certain enzymes break down endocannabinoids—the enzyme responsible for breaking down anandamide is called fatty acid amide hydrolase (FAAH). CBD, however, inhibits this enzyme, causing the levels of anandamide in the body to increase.

Endocannabinoids travel in a different direction to other neurotransmitters, known as "retrograde transmission", which is a contributing factor in their singular effects in the body. The term modulator is used with anandamide and other endocannabinoids because they change the flow of other neurotransmitters and thus impact upon how all other body systems and the brain operate.

Anandamide has a wide variety of effects in the body, and because the CB-1 and CB-2 receptors are so prolific, it is possible that anandamide has even more effects upon the body that have not yet been discovered. Thus far it is known that anandamide affects reproduction and fertility, reward, cell regulation, appetite regulation, pain relief, and mood. Current research has only discovered and named a handful of endocannabinoids, but it is thought there are more, and research is continuously ongoing.

The role of anandamide

Pain relief

Because of its "retrograde transmission", scientists believe that one of the primary functions of anandamide is pain modulation. Research has found that anandamide has analgesic effects because it modulates the TRPV-1 receptors which control pain.

Reward

Mostly, when we discuss the brain's reward mechanisms people think of dopamine—the "pleasure hormone". In actual fact, dopamine operates both as a neurotransmitter and a hormone and is activated by the TRPV-1 receptors which are modulated by anandamide. The brain has "reward pathways" which contain many dopamine neurons, but these reward path[1]ways also contain cannabinoid receptors and endocannabinoids, among them anandamide. Anandamide is thought to also stimulate hunger and the desire to eat, thus playing a part in appetite regulation. This has caused scientists to surmise that anandamide plays an important role in reward and pleasure.

The "runner's high"

It is a well-known adage—a healthy mind equals a healthy body, and it is also known that exercise "raises endorphins and boosts mood" which causes what is known as the "runner's high". This is described as a sudden burst of euphoria, analgesia, and mild sedation. A study performed in 2015 discovered that endocannabinoids, which included anandamide, were "crucial" to this "runner's high". A study published in the 2004 *Journal of Sports Medicine* posited that it is not in fact endorphins which create this feeling of euphoria, but has always been endocannabinoids—these were simply not well enough researched. Issues around being able to replicate "the runner's high" in a laboratory setting, and the fact that endorphins are too large to cross the blood–brain barrier and can therefore not be measured in the blood of an athlete after exercise, caused researchers to look at what else was in the athlete's blood. Increased quantities of anandamide were found, and this has prompted the hypothesis that it is in fact anandamide causing this euphoric feeling.

Mood enhancement

The endocannabinoid system is involved with mood and emotional regulation and cannabinoid receptors are to be found in significant areas of the brain which relate to these functions.

It is thought that anandamide helps to reduce anxiety and depression. In 2014 a study discovered that mice which were deficient in anandamide experienced more anxiety in response to stress, whereas those with higher levels of anandamide were far more able to cope. In a 2016 study, mouse models with diabetes and depression were found to have their symptoms reversed when their anandamide was increased. This has led scientists to posit that a deficiency in endocannabinoids may well induce depression and anxiety.

Reproduction and fertility

As it is believed that anandamide regulates hormones, sperm, and eggs within the reproductive system, it is thought that anandamide plays an important role in both male and female fertility and reproduction. A review published in 2014 concluded that anandamide could be used as a biomarker or indicator of infertility. If anandamide function is normal, this will predict normal fertility, whereas abnormalities in anandamide function appear to predict infertility.

Breast milk

A 2004 study published in the *European Journal of Pharmacology* suggested that endocannabinoids have a significant role to play in pre- and post-natal development. Endocannabinoids such as anandamide are found in both bovine (cow) and human breast milk. CB-1 receptors were seen to form before fourteen weeks of gestation, and it is thought that the endocannabinoid system is a fundamental factor in the development of a newborn's ability and desire to feed. Not only do these endocannabinoids have an appetite function, it has also been found that they help to protect neurons in the post-natal development of the brain. Another endocannabinoid found in significant quantities in human breast milk is 2-AG, which helps to mediate the immune system, hence the "breast is best" theory, as formula milk does not contain any cannabinoids.

Cell regulation and development

During the development of an embryo, stem cells differentiate into a variety of different cells which include brain, heart, and skin cells. It is thought that anandamide plays a significant role in the differentiation of brain cells into specific kinds of neurons during development.

Cell death, known as apoptosis, is a completely normal process undergone by damaged cells. This is a process which may take place when a cell is cancerous; it is the body's own defence mechanism to help prevent the spread of cancer. A study published in 2000 showed that anandamide triggered apoptosis in cancerous cells via the TRPV-1 receptors (also known as vanilloid receptors). It was discovered that human neuroblastoma and lymphoma cancer cells were more likely to die when there was more anandamide present, and less likely to die if anandamide was blocked.

Is it possible to increase anandamide?

Although anandamide is found naturally within the body, it is also possible to boost the amount of anandamide the body has.

A study conducted in 2012 discovered that cardiovascular exercise increased the levels of anandamide in the body; exercising therefore is an exceptionally good way to increase the body's levels.

Chocolate essentially contains low levels of anandamide, so the consumption of chocolate can also increase the body's levels of anandamide. Obviously, this should be good quality chocolate. Raw organic chocolate or cacao are probably the best ways to do this.

As discussed in the opening section about anandamide, CBD inhibits the enzyme responsible for breaking down anandamide—FAAH (fatty acid amide hydrolase). FAAH breaks down anandamide soon after it is released, but if it is inhibited, the anandamide stays in the body for longer with good effect; therefore using a CBD product will enhance how long anandamide stays within the body and can be extremely beneficial.

What is CBN? (cannabinol)

CBN, which is an abbreviation for cannabinol, is a mildly psychoactive cannabinoid which is, however, only found in trace amounts in cannabis. It is closely related to THC and is regulated as a controlled substance in the UK. CBN is formed as a metabolite of tetrahydrocannabinol (THC). It is formed when cannabis is exposed to air or sunlight for a significant amount of time, and thereby degraded, THC-A—the precursor to THC—is converted into cannabinolic acid (CBNA) and if this is decarboxylated (heated) it forms CBN. It is a partial agonist to CB-1 receptors but has more affinity with CB-2 receptors and works as an immunosuppressant or immunomodulator.

This has caused scientists to consider that CBN could be useful in conditions which involve an over-functioning immune system and could be beneficial in cases of Crohn's disease or arthritis. It could turn out to be a genuinely safer alternative for immunosuppression; obviously, research is still ongoing into this field.

- A 1995 study indicated that CBN can help induce sleep and lower body temperature, much like THC. The research published suggested CBN as an applicable cannabinoid to assist insomnia patients.
- In 2008, a study revealed that CBN showed potent activity against a variety of MRSA strains, thus displaying its potential antibacterial properties.

Cannabinol is a by-product of the degradation of cannabis. In other words, CBN tends to be in higher concentrations in medical cannabis that has not been stored properly. This means that to utilise CBN, one must leave the cannabis plant exposed for a period of time, allowing for more cannabinol and therefore less THC.

What is CBG? (cannabigerol)

CBG, also known as cannabigerol, is what has been considered a minor compound found within cannabis; it is the non-acidic form of cannabigerolic acid, which is considered to be the parent molecule from which other metabolites are formed, most notably THC and CBD during the growth cycle of the plant. Only a tiny amount of CBG is left in the plant, perhaps 1% at the end of its growth cycle; however, it is thought to have antibacterial and anti-inflammatory effects as well as promoting bone growth and inhibitory effects upon the growth of tumorous or cancerous cells. Cannabigerol is non-psychotropic, meaning it does not have the psychoactive effects in the way THC does.

CBG has until recently been completely overlooked, as it is found in such tiny quantities within the cannabis plant and thus was perceived to have little therapeutic benefit. Israeli scientists first isolated CBG during the 1960s at around the same time as THC; however, CBG has no psychoactive effects. It binds primarily to CB-2 receptors and research indicates that it may have significant anti-inflammatory effects.

Interestingly, very recent research has discovered that, although CBG is not thought to be highly prevalent within the cannabis plant, it is the likely stem cell or template for CBD and THC which means that in infancy both THC and CBD start out as cannabigerol. CBG is found in higher quantities in hemp strains rather than cannabis strains.

It has also been discovered that CBG inhibits the uptake of GABA, causing the feeling of relaxation which is normally associated with CBD. These discoveries have resulted in new and current interest in cannabigerol and it is hoped that new research may have more wide-reaching implications.

- A study published in *Neurotherapeutics* in 2015 discovered that CBG was enormously active as a neuroprotectant in mouse models with Huntingdon's disease. CBG improved motor deficits and preserved striatal neurons against toxicity. It also diminished the up-regulation of pro-inflammatory markers and improved levels of antioxidant defences. The study concluded that CBG showed a promising profile for some modest improvements in Huntingdon's disease; the researchers felt that perhaps in combination with other cannabinoids this could be improved upon significantly and urged for further research to take place.

- A study performed in 2014 found that CBG could protect from inflammation of the brain and spinal cord (autoimmune encephalomyelitis) as it has immunosuppressive qualities and suggested that this could have potential as a therapeutic agent for the treatment of inflammatory and autoimmune conditions.
- A study on colon cancer performed in 2014 discovered that cannabigerol could protect against colon tumours. Cell growth in colorectal cancer cells was evaluated and the study concluded that CBG "hampers colon cancer progression in vivo and selectively inhibits the growth of CRC cells", and also that "In vivo, CBG inhibited the growth of xenograft tumours as well as chemically induced colon carcinogenesis." Their findings concluded that cannabigerol should be considered in the prevention and potential cure of colorectal cancer.

What is CBDV? (cannabidivarin)

Cannabidivarin, also known as CBDV, is a non-psychoactive cannabinoid found in minor amounts in the hemp plant *Cannabis sativa*. A recently discovered cannabinoid, CBDV has been the subject of much research into its potential therapeutic properties.

GW Pharmaceuticals, the British company, collaborated with the University of Reading to perform a study which strongly suggested that cannabidivarin suppressed seizures in six different experimental models commonly used in epilepsy drug discovery. There are countless studies on CBDV and its anti-convulsant effects, specifically on epilepsy. GW Pharmaceuticals has now manufactured a product named "Epidiolex" approved by the FDA available in the United States for the treatment of Dravet's syndrome and Lennox-Gastaut syndrome, both rare and usually virtually untreatable types of epilepsy.

What is CBC? (cannabichromene)

Cannabichromene (abbreviated to CBC) is one of the lesser-known cannabinoids but it has its stem in cannabigerolic acid (CBGa); it is converted into cannabichrome carboxylic acid (CBCa) and then through an enzymatic process over time, or if exposed to heat (decarboxylation) the CBCa breaks down to become cannabichromene. This can happen with degradation and time not always requiring decarboxylation to take place. Interestingly, it is only tropical forms of cannabis which contain CBC and only in minute quantities, which makes it difficult to obtain. However, in research it has been found to have antimicrobial, antiviral, anti-inflammatory, antidepressant, analgesic, antiproliferative, and brain growth stimulating properties.

There has been some success in using CBC in the treatment of migraines. CBC inhibits the uptake of anandamide allowing it to stay in the bloodstream for longer, and thus has been shown to inhibit the growth of cancerous tumours particularly in human breast cancer. However, more research into the compound may be needed before any definitive medical effects can be verified.

- Studies have shown that CBC reduced inflammation, specifically in the intestinal tract. Unusually, CBC reduced inflammation without binding onto cannabinoid receptors in the patient's body, which has led to the theory that the combination of CBC with other cannabinoids that do latch onto receptors could be of significant medical value.
- A study published in 1981 tested the anti-inflammatory, antibacterial and antifungal activity of cannabichromene (CBC) and found it was superior to pharmacological drugs in antibacterial activity and had moderate antifungal activity. Its effects on *E.coli* and *Staphylococcus* were considered significant.
- A report published in 2013 found that cannabichromene could be helpful in neurological development, in particular neurogenesis. New research has discovered that neurogenesis does not only occur during foetal development but in fact continues in adult mammals in the hippocampus region of the brain. This is an area which is linked to information retention and memories. Associations with conditions such as Alzheimer's disease in the hippocampus region lead researchers to think that cannabichromene and its neurogenesis of this region of the brain could offer a viable treatment to ameliorate Alzheimer's and similar neurodegenerative diseases.
- In 2011 the *British Journal of Pharmacology* published a study inferring that CBC alleviated pain in test animals. This was not as profound or effective as the pain relief provided by THC; however, as cannabichromene is completely

non-psychoactive this could make it a viable and useful product for long-term pain relief.
- A study by the University of Mississippi identified CBC to have relatively strong antidepressant properties. However, the study could not verify how CBC releases these properties on the body, since it does not interact with the brain in the same way as other antidepressive cannabinoids (THC).

What is THCV? (tetrahydrocannabivarin)

Tetrahydrocannabivarin (THCV) is structurally almost identical to tetrahydrocannabinol (THC) although its formation is entirely different and there are significant variances in the effects of the compound.

Instead of starting its embryonic life as cannabigerolic acid (CBGa), geranyl pyrophosphate combines with divarinolic acid resulting in cannabigerovarin acid (CBGVA).

Once CBGVA has been created the development process of THCV continues along the same path as THC. CBGVA is broken down to tetrahydrocannabivarin carboxylic acid (THCVA) and can then be decarboxylated with heat or light to create THCV.

Both THC and THCV affect the same receptors, but in a slightly different manner.

- The neurology department of Aberdeen University has carried out studies on THCV with regard to its appetite

suppressant properties. Results indicate that THCV is ideal for conditions where weight loss is necessary.
- Owing to its appetite suppressant properties, THCV is unsuitable for those persons suffering from cachexia, anorexia, and other similar conditions. THCV also has a different boiling point to THC (220 degrees Celsius) meaning that patients using vaporising as a method of ingestion will need to heat their product to a higher temperature.
- In small doses THCV appears to have no psychoactive effect; however, in high doses, it is known to produce a very intense euphoric psychoactive effect and must be carefully administered. It has been discovered that the psychoactive effects, while significantly stronger than THC, last approximately half the time. Some Israeli research has indicated that THCV could alleviate panic attacks in patients suffering from post-traumatic stress disorder. Interestingly, it does not suppress other emotions, selectively only suppressing the ability to panic associated with acute stress responses.
- Research indicates that THCV could stimulate bone growth and research is ongoing regarding its potential in the treatment of osteoporosis and other degenerative bone diseases.
- Research into the relationship between THCV and tremors associated with Parkinson's has suggested a significant reduction in erratic, uncontrolled movement.
- Studies suggest that THCV has the ability to regulate blood sugar levels, with significant research into its link with the treatment of diabetes now underway. GW Pharmaceuticals is at the forefront of this research, attempting to develop an alternative to metformin using THCV.

CHAPTER 4

The endocannabinoid system

The endocannabinoid system is the crux to why cannabis has become such a valuable and effective tool. Every living being has an endocannabinoid system, but no one considers it when looking at anatomy and physiology—it is not taught in most medical schools and was only discovered in 1988 making it still a very new discovery which needs to be learnt about. I often joke when I talk to my patients about the endocannabinoid system using my favourite "Lord of the Rings" reference—it is the "one to rule them all" as it has receptors and therefore affects every single body organ including the brain.

Every living being has an endocannabinoid system, including mammals, birds, reptiles, and fish. Even amphibians seem to have a primitive version. The system is not exactly the same in all creatures, so we will concentrate on the human endocannabinoid system—which is, however, much the same in all mammals, including your pet dog or cat.

The Israeli scientist, Dr Raphael Mechoulam at the Hebrew University of Jerusalem, isolated THC in 1964 and he is often hailed as "the man" within cannabis communities, although there is evidence that THC was already discovered in 1940 by a scientist from the United States named Adams. Nevertheless, Mechoulam has continued and done some incredibly important research with regards to the isolation of THC and other cannabinoids. In 1988 an American scientist (Allyn C Howlett) discovered the cannabinoid receptor—by using a radioactive dye attached to synthetic THC it was noted whereabouts the THC went in the brain and saw that it selectively attached to a specific receptor.

The puzzling factor was, why would THC attach to a specific receptor and why did the body contain this receptor in the first place? The theory was that the body must produce its own type of cannabis to lock into this specific receptor. The first of these was not discovered until 1992 and it was in fact N-arachidonoylethanolamine or AEA—more popularly termed "anandamide". In 1995 a further compound was discovered and called 2-arachidonylglylycerol or 2-AG. These two substances were regarded as "endogenous cannabinoids" or "endocannabinoids" for short. A further cannabis receptor was then discovered within the immune system and interest in the potential "endocannabinoid system" exploded.

Endocannabinoids are effectively fatty substances or oils in microscopic quantities which interact or bind with cannabinoid receptors in a lock and key type system. Cannabinoid receptors are membranes in the body's cells that enable signals to be passed back and forth. There are CB-1 and CB-2 receptors in the immune and gastrointestinal system (see Chapter 5).

There are enzymes that synthesise and degrade the endocannabinoids such as fatty acid amide or monoacylglycerol lipase. The human body manufactures endocannabinoids in order to pass messages concerning functions such as pain, inflammation, memory, appetite, and mood. CBD is a phytocannabinoid that interacts with the cannabinoid receptors found in the body. Most phytocannabinoids are from the cannabis plant although some other plants such as echinacea and hops also contain cannabinoid-like substances.

Phytocannabinoids such as CBD can affect the body in the same way as endocannabinoids. It follows that phytocannabinoids can affect pain, inflammation, memory, appetite, and mood.

The endocannabinoid system is a regulatory internal system to manage the signals sent between cells within the body with the aim of maintaining balance or homeostasis. Effectively what will happen is that something in your body will trigger a response to create the endocannabinoid—and that trigger might be pain, inflammation, an injury, or other "dis-ease". The body is like a machine that always seeks to be in balance, and when a stressor affects the body creating an imbalance the body, like a child's mobile, tries to rebalance what it perceives as an anomaly.

Imagine a child's mobile—it has lots of different things hanging and spinning gently, always balanced. However, if you tug on one of the items, the whole thing loses its shape and becomes unbalanced—the body is almost identical. Stress for example, raises adrenaline, which in turn raises cortisol levels, destabilising insulin, and frequently thereby disturbing thyroid hormones and sex hormones—the whole system is slightly out of kilter. Endocannabinoids are released by cells in response to such a trigger and the endocannabinoid system will determine how the body needs to be balanced.

The endocannabinoid system has receptors in every single body system and thus helps to balance:

- The immune system
- Digestion
- The cardiovascular system
- Mental health
- Eye health and intraocular pressure
- Hormonal regulation
- Maintenance of bone mass
- Pain perception
- Metabolic control
- Inflammatory reactions

- Memory
- Appetite
- Skin health
- Neuronal protection
- Reward circuits

This really does show how the endocannabinoid system is the "one to rule them all" because it appears to be involved in almost every chemical process within the body.

If there is a failure in the endocannabinoid system, it will result in a serious imbalance which will have repercussions on every single organ system. A disruption to the endocannabinoid system can occur owing to the body's need to try to balance by manufacturing more or less endocannabinoids in response to a stressor.

Each human being's endocannabinoid system is also different—different patients show different responses to cannabis medicines despite using identical products. There is a genetic difference in different people in how the baseline endocannabinoid system function works. If someone has an imbalance in their endocannabinoid system, they may experience a completely different reaction or result with the type of cannabis medication they use. This was underlined to me recently with a situation where my foster son started sneezing after eating some 80% cacao dark chocolate. He complained that he always sneezes after eating dark chocolate and so do several members of his family. I researched "allergy to dark chocolate" and found that a large number of people sneeze when eating dark chocolate—this is because of a genetic predisposition going back to Neanderthal genes—thus genes can predispose a person to being more or less sensitive to chocolate, and so it is also with cannabinoids.

As a foster carer for twenty years, I was very used to looking after children with ADHD and ADD typical behaviour. These children respond very differently to stimuli than other children and are often given stimulants to calm their brains down, such as Ritalin. What would make a non-ADHD person very hyperactive actually calms down the hyperactive person—because they have a different set of neurotransmitters which fire differently. The same is true of many patients using medical cannabis: variations in genetic code, neurotransmitters, and how each person is made up will alter how cannabis medication works on them. I often tell patients that not everyone can tolerate paracetamol or anti-inflammatories—it is basically the same concept.

Our bodies are made to adapt to situations and conditions, and so they do. The point of being a medical herbalist is to get to the root cause of such conditions and treat the organ system that is considered to be faulty after examining all the evidence during a thorough consultation.

Balancing the endocannabinoid system

The endocannabinoid system is extremely complex and because it has receptors in every organ system, the way to look at how to balance it is to consider how it might have become unbalanced in the first place. There are several things that can cause the endocannabinoid system to become unbalanced.

Stress response

My professor at university had his favourite analogy when discussing stress. You are wandering down the high street in your local town, when suddenly a tiger leaps out at you. Your body is designed to deal with this, with its fight or flight response. The amygdala (a segment within the brain often called "the emotional brain") senses danger and makes a split second decision to initiate the fight or flight response before your "thinking brain" the neocortex, has time to react. This response immediately decides what to do, whether it feels you are capable of turning and facing and fighting the tiger, or whether you should run away. The stress response causes adrenaline to surge, preparing you for flight. However, the unconscious part of the brain that is responsible for such responses doesn't differentiate particularly well between "tiger in high street" and "parking warden giving you a ticket" or "the washing machine breaking down" or "your boss giving you a deadline at work". The body still responds with its primordial response of fight or flight. Whilst on an evolutionary level we may have had to deal with physical threats upon which our survival depended, our lizard brain does not differentiate subtleties of threat level. The subtle stresses we deal with on a daily basis nowadays are still reacted to in the same way by the amygdala. Adrenaline surges, cortisol rises, insulin becomes unbalanced and *all* of this is controlled from below by the endocannabinoid system which causes anandamide (the feel-good endocannabinoid) to be reduced, with increased levels of 2-AG thus reducing the perception of pain. As these daily life stresses continue the body has to adapt to the fact that it cannot escape from the figurative tiger (or boss/husband/wife/traffic warden), and having constantly high levels of 2-AG overstimulates CB-1 receptors in the brain and thus the brain responds by decreasing its CB-1 receptors.

It is like a domino effect: there are now fewer endocannabinoid receptors in the brain and emotional balance becomes difficult to maintain, causing low mood and ultimately depression.

Dietary response

Since the 1960s, our diet has changed. We are eating more processed, packaged, ready to consume, high carbohydrate and sugar-laden foods than ever before—and we have an upsurge in autoimmune conditions—there must be a correlation.

As discussed in the description of the different cannabinoids, the endocannabinoid system controls the appetite.

By eating a diet rich in sugars, carbohydrates, and processed foods, there is an increase of endocannabinoids in the intestine and circulatory system, which has the result of making the person hungrier and thus eating more and the whole thing becomes a vicious circle. Fat cells produce more endocannabinoids which make the patient even more hungry. This in turn leads to extra weight which puts pressure onto the joints, and invariably causes painful conditions.

Drugs and alcohol

Research is beginning to show that the long-term use of recreational and pharmaceutical drugs is having an effect on the endocannabinoid system. Overstimulating endocannabinoid receptors with regular use of drugs, alcohol, and pharmaceuticals can lead over time to a tolerance effect which causes the CB-1 receptors to become down-regulated in the brain. Some studies have suggested that when an alcoholic goes into withdrawal the CB-1 receptors will initially reduce and it may take weeks or more to return to normal levels. The results of trials reveal a "critical role for CB-1 receptors in clinically important aspects of alcohol dependence and provide a rationale for the use of CB-1 receptor antagonists in the treatment of addiction".

Genetic predisposition

Because DNA is so complex, there are millions of areas where the blueprint for neurotransmitter development diverges—which explains why the endocannabinoid system is so different in each individual.

Restoring the balance

The consumption of cannabis-based products will mimic the body's own endocannabinoid system and may help to restore balance. However, this is in some ways a reductionist approach. The entire approach needs to be far more holistic.

As discussed during the section on anandamide, the euphoria that a person feels known as "the runner's high" means that exercise is a great way to restore balance in the endocannabinoid system. An hour or more of moderate exercise can raise blood levels of anandamide and the effect will bring about a temporary reduction in pain levels, can reduce anxiety levels, and not only increase the body's anandamide levels but also the levels of 2-AG, boosting mood and helping to maintain a healthy weight and manage stress levels.

Phytocannabinoids

Cannabinoids which can be found in other plants may also help boost the endocannabinoid system. Cacao, as mentioned previously (and therefore good quality chocolate rich in cacao), is only one of these. Others include maca, black pepper, nutmeg, black truffles, ginger, hops, broccoli, cauliflower, cabbage, brussels sprouts, carrots, celery, parsley, and herbs such as echinacea, *Helichrysum umbraculigerum*, liverwort (*Radula marginata*), kava (*Piper methysticum*), and *Panax ginseng*— amongst others.

CBD and its interaction with the endocannabinoid system

Obviously cannabidiol (CBD) is also a phytocannabinoid; however, it behaves slightly differently to other phytocannabinoids such as THC. It does not stimulate the endocannabinoid system in the same way as THC—which poses a risk of overstimulation; instead, it modifies the CB-1 receptors making them less likely to activate or over-activate. CBD also enhances the boosting of endocannabinoids by inhibiting re-uptake and degradation. As CBD meets both aspects of activity upon the endocannabinoid system this creates a balancing effect and can be a valuable outcome for the user. The pleiotropy and promiscuity of the cannabinoids mean that CBD binds to more than one type of receptor. It has a significant effect upon the serotonergic system. However, the endocannabinoid system is not the only system affected by CBD; it also has positive effects upon opioid receptors and dopamine receptors among many others.

The biphasic effect

What does "biphasic" mean? In general terms, a biphasic drug is one that has different effects upon the body at varying blood concentration levels.

Cannabinoids have "biphasic properties". For simplification purposes—it is known that alcohol has "biphasic properties", whilst a low dose of alcohol can act as a stimulant, at a high dose it will have a depressive or sedative effect on the body. Caffeine has similar biphasic properties.

To make it easier to understand CBD and how it might work with a patient it is vital to consider the biphasic response of CBD. I have seen many patients who think that if one drop is good for you, two must be better, and ten must be great. In the shop where I used to work people were always coming in and asking for "the strongest thing you've got" because their condition felt so severe to them that they wanted to go straight in at the strongest level. This is not the case with CBD—less is more, as I have found myself telling patients and other practitioners very regularly.

CBD interacts with the endocannabinoid system and when this is in a minute, low dose, this can increase alertness, energy levels, wakefulness, and many other uplifting responses. When CBD is administered in higher-level doses, however, it has a sedating effect. It is noticeable when someone is using too much CBD as they will feel much sleepier and calm rather than energetic and alert.

Because of the biphasic properties of cannabis, it has a vast array of applications in practice, from insomnia to chronic pain. However, this biphasic effect means it is extremely important to start almost every patient off on an extremely low dose of CBD, and then very gradually increase it drop by drop over several weeks if necessary. I always recommend at least a week to ten days before increasing the amount of product the patient is taking. If they start on too high a dose, it is likely the CBD will have an opposite effect to the one they are hoping for. It is also possible that the CBD will react to the endocannabinoid system by "closing receptors" because the system has been flooded, and then the product will be excreted without any effects upon the body whatsoever. Another side effect of taking too much CBD too quickly could be what is known as the "Herxheimer reaction".

The Herxheimer reaction

The Herxheimer reaction is also known as "Herxing" and it short term reaction by the body as the body is detoxified. It is possible to experience flu-like symptoms including such conditions as a headache, joint and muscle pain, body aches, a sore throat, chills, nausea, or sweating. This effect can last for several days, a week or even more. Herxing is not unique to CBD; it can happen with other herbs or pharmaceuticals also; it is something my university professor used to call an "abreaction" or a "defence reaction". The body does not recognise the large amount of whatever is being ingested and produces a defence effect to try to ameliorate this.

Herxheimer's reaction was initially noted in the treatment of syphilis with strong antibiotics. Traditionally known as the Jarisch–Herxheimer reaction it was described by two physicians in different time periods: Dr Adolf Jarish (1860–1902) from Vienna, Austria, and some years later by Dr Karl Herxheimer (1861–1942) who was from Frankfurt,

Germany. Both physicians noted a bizarre reaction while treating syphilitic lesions of the skin. Their research noted that in response to certain strong treatments patients experienced a worsening of their symptoms to a significant level before the condition settled down and healed.

By using a "low and slow" regimen of CBD it is possible to reduce the likelihood of a Herxheimer reaction.

CHAPTER 5

The CB-1 and CB-2 receptors

THE ENDOCANNABINOID SYSTEM
CANNABINOID RECEPTORS

 CB1 - Receptors are concentrated in the brain and the central nervous system but are also present in some nerves and organs

 CB2 - Receptors are predominantly in peripheral organs, particularly in cells associated with the immune system.

 TRVP1 - Receptors are found most prolifically in the blood, bone marrow, tongue, kidney, liver, stomach and ovaries.

 TRVP2 - Receptors are concentrated in the skin, muscle, kidney, stomach and lungs.

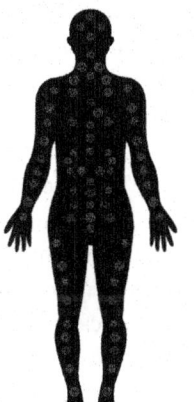

 GPR55 - Receptors are found in the bones, the brain, especially in the cerebellum, and in the jejunum and ileum within the GI tract.

 GPR18 - Receptors are primarily found within bone marrow, the spleen and lymph nodes and to a lesser extent in the testes.

 GPR119 - Receptors are found predominantly in the pancreas and the intestinal tract, in small amounts.

What are CB-1 receptors?

Cannabinoid receptor type 1 (CB-1) is a G protein-coupled cannabinoid receptor found predominantly in the peripheral and central nervous systems. It was only discovered in the late 1980s and assists with a variety of functions in the body which include controlling brain activity, regulating the immune system, and stabilising heart conditions, among many others. The body produces its own cannabinoids, as discussed previously, within the "endogenous cannabinoid system" or "endocannabinoid system". Current research also posits that there may well be other cannabinoid receptors in the human body (GPR18, GPR55, and GPR119) although research is still ongoing, and these have not yet been formally analysed and named.

CB-1 receptors are concentrated predominantly in the brain and central nervous system although they also sporadically populate other areas of the body. These are activated not only by the body's own endocannabinoids such as anandamide and AG-2, but also through phytocannabinoids which are introduced to the body such as CBD or THC.

Research has been ongoing for the past two decades and numerous studies have implicated CB-1 receptors as an important factor in internal health maintenance. Studies indicate that active CB-1 receptors moderate neurotransmitter releases in a way that manages disproportionate neuronal activity and thereby alleviates pain and inflammation. This revelation is crucial when considering the discovery that CB-1 receptors are found in elevated quantities in carcinoma tumour samples and other human prostate cancer cells. This has caused scientists to posit that active CB-1 receptors could be vital to the prevention of growth and inflammation of cancer cells.

A 2015 study which concentrated on investigating the depressive behavioural tendencies of mice, discovered that CB-1 receptors have antidepressant effects when enacted with endocannabinoids. The outcomes gave clear proof that the endo-cannabinoid framework assumes a key role in controlling such tendencies.

A critical analysis published in November 2020 has suggested that the CB-1 allosteric modulators could have potential in the treatment of central nervous system disorders. The paper discussed that novel strategies are under investigation targeting CB-1 with emphasis on "the elimination or mitigation of potential psychiatric adverse effects observed by central agonism/antagonism of CB-1". Research is underway to avoid the adverse effects while maintaining the therapeutic benefits of modulating CB-1.

What are CB-2 receptors?

During the early 1990s Cambridge University researchers seeking a second receptor which could explain the therapeutic properties of cannabis discovered the cannabinoid receptor type 2, abbreviated as CB-2. This is a G protein-coupled receptor encoded within the CNR2 (cannabinoid receptor 2) gene and is closely related to its cannabinoid receptor type 1 (CB-1) counterpart. The principal endogenous ligand for the CB-2 receptor is 2-arachidonylglycerol or 2-AG. Discovery of this receptor played a vital role in studying the endocannabinoid system and its effects upon the immune system.

Despite the close affinity to their CB-1 counterparts, CB-2 receptors do not transmit as efficiently to the brain as CB-1 receptors, although they have still been known to play a role in modulating neurological disorders. Instead, CB-2 receptors are concentrated predominantly in peripheral organs, most commonly the immune system, the gastrointestinal system, and the peripheral nervous system.

Scientific studies have determined that CB-2 receptors are prolific throughout tissues of the immune system. These receptors have shown regulatory action upon the release of cytokines, the proteins that control development and responsiveness of those cells that respond to infection or inflammation.

The peripheral nervous system has also been shown to have such CB-2 receptors wherein they are able to propitiate valuable effects. One of the most significant discoveries with regard to the function of CB-2 receptors is their management and control of inflammation in the gastrointestinal system, which could lead to exciting future options with regard to controlling gastrointestinal diseases such as Crohn's disease or irritable bowel syndrome.

While CB-1 receptors are far more prevalent and important in the role of brain function, CB-2 receptors have nevertheless been discovered within the brain. The main difference in their mode of action is that whereas CB-1 receptors work congruently with neurons, CB-2 receptors work specifically with microglia cells. Microglia cells have a wide variety of functions. They are the primary immune cells of the central nervous system and respond to pathogens and injury by changing the morphology and migrating to the site of infection or injury where they destroy pathogens and remove damaged cells in a similar way to peripheral macrophages.

CHAPTER 6

Metabolism

The endocannabinoid system and homeostasis

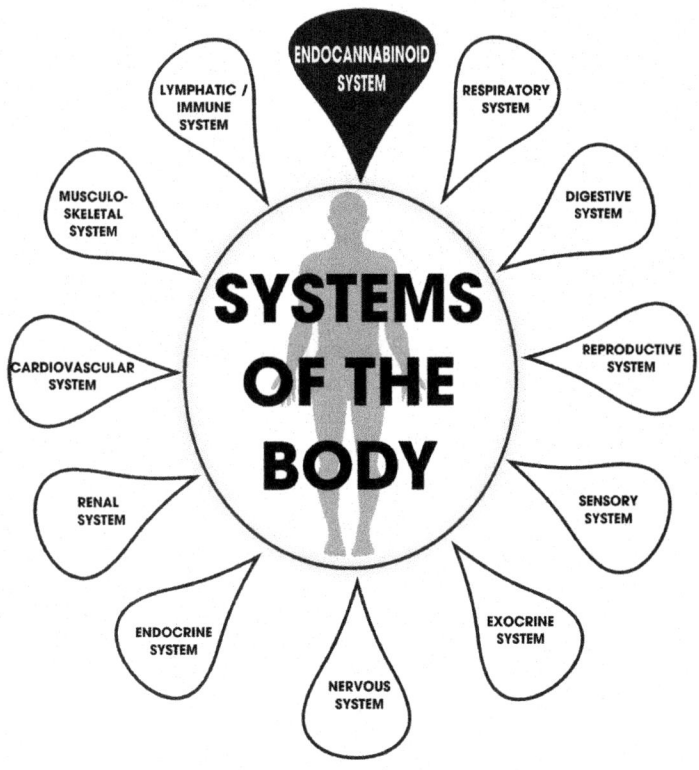

During lectures, this is one of my favourite diagrams as it is the introduction to my "one to rule them all" analogy. As you can see the endocannabinoid system affects and balances every single other body system. If the endocannabinoid system is out of alignment, or unbalanced, there will be no stability or homeostasis.

An abstract from the 2007 paper on "The role of the endocannabinoid system in the regulation of endocrine function and in the control of energy balance in humans" by Jan Komorowski and Henryk Stepien is enlightening and is shared in its entirety, below:

> The endocannabinoid system has been recently recognised as an important modulatory system in the function of the brain, endocrine, and immune tissues. It appears to play a particularly important regulatory role in the secretion of hormones related to reproductive functions and response to stress. The important elements of this system are endocannabinoid receptors (types CB-1 and CB-2), their endogenous ligands (N-arachidonoylethanolamide, 2-arachidonoyl glycerol), enzymes involved in their synthesis and degradation, as well as cannabinoid antagonists.
>
> In humans this system also controls energy homeostasis and mainly influences the function of the food intake centres of the central nervous system and gastrointestinal tract activity. The endocannabinoid system regulates not only the central and peripheral mechanisms of food intake, but also lipids synthesis and turnover in the liver and adipose tissue as well as glucose metabolism in muscle cells. Rimonabant, a new and selective central and peripheral cannabinoid-1 receptor (CB-1) blocker, has been shown to reduce body weight and improve cardiovascular risk factor (metabolic syndrome) in obese patients by increasing HDL-cholesterol and adiponectin blood levels as well as

decreasing LDL-cholesterol, leptin, and C-reactive protein (a pro-inflammatory marker) concentrations.

It is therefore possible to speculate about a future clinical use of CB-1 antagonists, as a means of improving gonadotrophin pulsatility and fertilisation capacity as well as the prevention of cardiovascular disease and type 2 diabetes mellitus. Drugs acting as agonists of CB-1 receptors (Dronabinol, Dexanabinol) are currently proposed for evaluation as drugs to treat neurodegenerative disorders (Alzheimer's and Parkinson's diseases), epilepsy, anxiety, and stroke.

Metabolisation and CYP450 interaction

Cannabidiol (CBD) is considered a safe compound which is non-addictive and does not cause intoxication. It appears to have substantial therapeutic qualities, yet CBD–drug interactions could be an issue in a few instances.

Metabolism is the conversion by the body of chemical compounds through proteins known as enzymes. Enzymes are naturally found in the body and they speed up chemical reactions, an action known as catalysation.

The liver has a family of enzymes named cytochrome P450 (CYP450) which is the key enzyme group that metabolises the majority of drugs, alcohol, and substances we consume—and that includes the pharmaceutical drugs as well as supplements.

Metabolism consists of two phases—first pass (1) and second pass (2). In the first pass, oxygen is added to the compound (oxidation) thereby losing electrons. Once this first pass (phase 1) is completed, substances are "oxidised". In the second pass (phase 2), the substance is made more water soluble to allow for extraction, and during this phase a compound will become more inactive, losing its pharmacological activity as it gradually leaves the body. To reiterate, as a compound enters the body, it is at its peak of chemical activity. As it goes through the phases and passes through the enzymes in the liver it begins to break down and becomes inactive and water soluble and is then excreted.

A drug or compound is therefore absorbed via the gastrointestinal tract and passes via the hepatic portal vein to the liver; this can mean that with ingested compounds only a proportion of the drug will reach circulation. It is for this reason that we would recommend taking for example, a pepper together with curcumin (turmeric) to "enhance bioavailability" and ensure that more of the active ingredient is circulated around the body.

The first pass happens predominantly in the gut and liver, so certain drugs such as insulin will be metabolised in the gut, whereas other drugs such as propranolol will be metabolised in the liver.

Cytochrome P450 (CYP) enzymes are monooxygenases which are bound to endoplasmic reticulum membranes or mitochondria within the body, including the liver, kidney, lung, intestine, brain, heart, and integumentary system. The highest concentration of these is within the liver and intestine.

The CYP450 subfamilies such as CYP3A, CYP2C, CYP2D, and CYP2B are crucial to the metabolism of chemical compounds introduced to the body. Substantial variability of effects is dependent upon a variety of factors and key processes within individual metabolisation as well as extrinsic factors. Thus, pharmacokinetically there can be a variance in response, and CYP activity is involved in the metabolism of endocannabinoids such as anandamide as well as cholesterol, bile acids, vitamin D, steroid hormones, and compounds involved in cellular activity.

CBD appears to have an inhibitory effect on metabolism, taking up the entire bandwidth of CYP450, so concomitant ingestion of CBD alongside other pharmaceuticals, and even some foods (such as garlic) will mean that the other compounds or chemicals will not be metabolised correctly, if at all. If the dose of the supplement is high enough, there could be a deactivation of CYP450 enzymes by CBD, which could alter the way the patient metabolises various compounds, including tetrahydrocannabinol (THC). As mentioned above, this can be variable in individuals and depends entirely upon how *their* body metabolises CBD.

THC metabolisation

As mentioned during the discussion on CB-1 and CB-2 receptors, tetrahydrocannabinol (THC) acts upon the CB-1 cannabinoid receptor in the brain which by its metabolisation creates a significant high, indicating that the body's own metabolisation of THC makes the THC more potent. By oxidising compounds, (adding an oxygen atom into a compound's molecular structure) the body, specifically cytochrome P450, makes compounds more water soluble and easier for kidney filtration.

By administering cannabis in different ways, there will be different effects. By inhaling THC (smoking) the compound passes into the capillaries of the lungs, and then into blood circulation through the pulmonary arteries, rapidly crossing the blood/brain barrier. However, if ingested orally (swallowed) the THC will be absorbed into the small intestine and then carried on to the liver, where subclasses of CYP450 (for example CYP2C and CYP3A) metabolise the compound within the liver.

Sublingual application of CBD, provided it is done properly, means that the CBD is absorbed into the mucous membranes and thus in trials there is evidence that it has no effect on CYP450. During clinical trials for GW Pharmaceuticals' "Sativex" product, it was found that even at 40 mg sublingual dose, there was no change to CYP450 pathways.

What does this mean for herb–drug interactions?

Having worked in a store that sold CBD products to the public every day, as well as contributing to an internet forum which gives advice to customers and patients who want to know what is the best product for them to use for specific conditions, I have found that the easiest thing to tell people is to leave a gap between taking CBD and *any* other compound. Some people are on no other medications; however, I will still stress that should they get a headache and take paracetamol or ibuprofen, they need to leave at least a two-hour gap between these and their CBD—so, for example, take all meds at 8 am—then take CBD at between 10 and 11 am. Always ensure there is a time lapse between taking one and the other, to allow CYP450 to do its work on the other compounds being metabolised, before it has to deal with CBD. Generally, I advise a two-hour gap between products; however, if the patient is taking morphine, for example, I will suggest a four-hour gap. This can often be difficult for people to manage, as they sometimes have to take medicines every four hours—in which case I would always prescribe an oil rather than capsules, as the oil, sublingually, absorbs into the bloodstream—avoiding the liver and its CYP450 group of enzymes, whereas capsules need to be ingested and go through the gut, so they will interact.

Interestingly with the current predilection for polypharmacy (multitudes of prescription drugs all taken at the same time), when one looks at a patient's prescription, it is evident that some of the drugs listed interact with each other negatively. It is surprising how many people will happily take garlic supplements, for example, which also metabolise through CYP450, and not give it a second thought.

CHAPTER 7

Indica or sativa — what is the difference?

The explanation of how different cannabis extracts work and why some are energising, cerebral, and enlivening and others are soporific, relaxing, and anxiolytic is often portrayed by the different plant chemotype that is used in the manufacture, whether it is indica or sativa. However, there is significant scientific debate upon this subject and according to some scientists words like sativa and indica are no longer reliable indicators of the content of the plant.

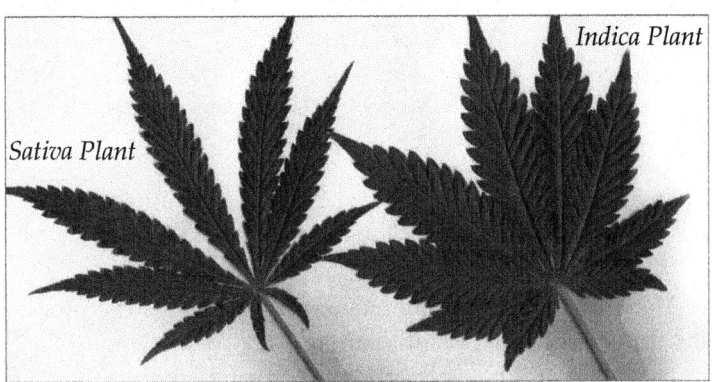

Originally indica and sativa described the plant morphology or physical attributes of the different strains of cannabis; however, prior to the farming and cross-breeding of cannabis strains to produce higher levels of THC and thus a more profitable drug yield for the recreational market there were probably only around sixty naturally evolving strains.

The sativa strains are long, tall, thin plants, evolved to survive in humid and hot environments. However, in hot dry climates short plants with broader leaves evolved which were discovered to have significant muscle relaxing properties. At this point in history—probably in the latter part of the nineteeth century, physical shape would have been an accurate predictor of chemical content and drug properties. However, in the twenty-first century, we now have over 6000 different hybridised strains, all based on the original sixty strains and as a result of this severe overbreeding the chemistry of the plant no longer bears any reliable relationship to its physical morphology.

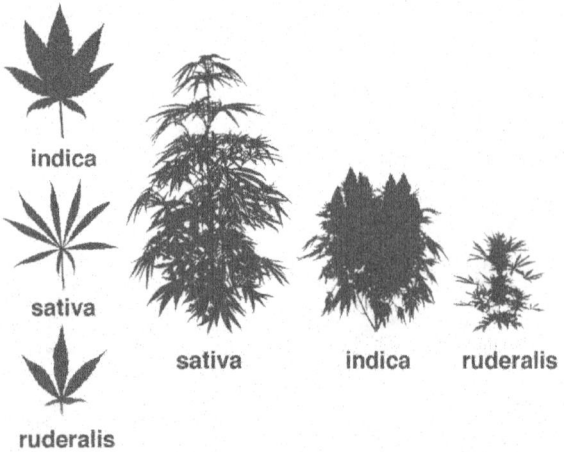

These days there is only one way to determine the properties of an individual plant accurately and reliably and that is through a thorough scientific component analysis in laboratory conditions. It is notable that the terpene profiles of certain plants confer those properties associated with sativa or indica plants. So a plant with more limonene for example would have more "sativa"—uplifting, energising effects than a plant with high levels of myrcene or beta-caryophyllene, which would give it more pain relieving, soporific, indica type effects.

It is highly likely that cannabis producers are labelling their products as indica and sativa based upon their effects rather than their scientific genetics. The labelling may still help consumers to find the product that works for them. There is also an issue in the UK that "indica" labelled products are not legally permitted. Their premise is that the only cannabis that is permitted to be imported and used for cannabidiol products should be hemp, sativa. This subject is hammered firmly home by the Cannabis Trade Association and the CLEAR Cannabis Law Reform group, but other references to this "law" are harder to find. As it is the higher levels of certain terpenes that confer the "indica" effect, it is possible to create "indica type" products, which have the properties of indica, even though they are created from a sativa plant.

Researchers who have considered the contrasts among indica and sativa have thought of various hypotheses dependent on hereditary qualities. The prevailing hypothesis centres upon the genetic production of THC and CBD.

Plants that produce abnormal amounts of THC express qualities that code for the compound THC-A synthase. This catalyst converts CBG into THC-A, which in turn converts into THC when decarboxylated (or heated). These plants are ordinarily considered indica.

Then again, a few plants express qualities that code for the compound CBDA synthase. This catalyst changes CBG into CBDA, the antecedent of CBD. These plants are commonly considered as being sativa.

As a result of these findings it is generally considered that indica plants have a higher THC:CBD ratio whereas sativa plants have a higher CBD:THC ratio. However, even scientists struggle to agree on this theory and there is disagreement with some claiming it is the other way around.

The issue is that, today, numerous strains produce differing measures of the two compounds. A number of scientists accept this is because of hybridisation of the gene pools, which clarifies why some salivas are rich in THC and some indicas are definitely not.

The anticipated effects of an "indica" or "sativa" strain of plant

In its original chemovar (chemically distinct variety), the sativa strain had energising, stimulating, cerebral, uplifting, creativity-enhancing, focusing, and anti-depressive qualities. By contrast, the indica strain had soporific, relaxing, sleep-inducing, pain-, stress-, anxiety-, and nausea-relieving properties.

This should help the person choosing to decide which product may be best for them. As outlined sativa strains are much more stimulating and indica strains far more sedating.

The energising, stimulating, and cerebral, mood uplifting effects of the sativa strains are very well suited to daytime use. A feeling of well-being and ease is often associated with sativa chemovars, making them ideal for social situations, to use whilst at work or if having to drive. They are said to promote deep conversation and enhance creativity.

Indica strains are far more soporific. They are much more suited to evening or night-time use as they can help a person to wind down and relax as well as relieving stress and aiding sleep.

All CBD products are anti-inflammatory—cannabis is renowned for its anti-inflammatory properties, so both sativa and indica chemovars will aid with the relief of inflammation. Generally, the indica chemovars will be better for painful conditions and sativa chemovars are better for depression and enhancing mental clarity; however, there are exceptions based on each individual's experience.

When I ran health stores, I would see hundreds of customers each week, and it was remarkable to notice how differently people reacted to the same products. The range of products I had available at that time consisted of sativa chemovars, indica chemovars, and also an indica dominant hybrid as well as a sativa dominant hybrid. With patients suffering from ADHD or extreme anxiety I soon found that an indica or indica hybrid product was working best at calming down the brain and stopping those panic attacks and episodes. Yet I have had patients who subsequently found they were more "wired" after taking the indica products than they are when taking the sativa products. I used to tell these people that they were "opposites"—their wiring was different. This is presumably down to each person's specific genetic make-up. An analogy for this, to me, is the different way that neurodiverse people react to medicines. That does not mean that every person who reacts as an "opposite" is neurodiverse, just that their genetic make-up is slightly different.

Whilst it is difficult to generalise because of the different genetic code of each person, and the resultant different outcomes on occasions with various different products, the following list should not be considered exclusive, and if one chemovar doesn't work for a person it is worth considering using another to see if that gives the required effect. However, on the whole, the conditions on the list appear to be helped most by the following chemovars.

Indica chemovar subtype

Conditions such as multiple sclerosis, glaucoma, chronic pain, Crohn's disease, and sleep disorders generally find an indica product most beneficial.

An indica subtype can also be used to treat anxiety, as many people find that a sativa chemovar can exacerbate anxiety or even create paranoia.

Sativa based products can also be used for moderate relief from the above types of conditions as some people will prefer having a daytime energy-boosting effect rather than the soporific effect.

Sativa chemovar subtype

Due to their energising and uplifting effects, sativa chemovars can be wonderful for people suffering from mood disorders and also hormonal imbalances such as menopausal issues. Some people with anxiety react well to these, but others find that certain strains may increase their anxiety levels, so it is considered best for people to test out a product before committing to a regime. As all CBD regardless of chemovar is anti-inflammatory, in practice I have found this type to work very well for people with fibromyalgia, polymyalgia rheumatica, arthritis, aching joints, sciatica, and other joint and muscular problems. Because fibromyalgia causes the well-known "fibrofog" where sufferers struggle to think clearly, a sativa chemovar can enhance mental clarity and I have found it particularly helpful in such cases.

Hybrid chemovars

Technically every product on the market today is a hybrid of some kind, as the original sixty plant varieties have been so overbred and hybridised. A hybrid of cannabis is a crossbreed of different strains that have both indica and sativa genetics. They can take after either parent or be a blend of both. The goal is usually to attempt to create a strain with desirable characteristics from both.

- Hybrids are relatively common, and many popular indica and sativa strains have hybridisation somewhere in their ancestry.
- In some cases, a hybrid strain may be more characteristic or dominant of one species (indica or sativa).

- Hybridisation, also known as crossbreeding, can be useful for many different reasons.
- Growers consider indica, with its six- to eight-week maturation time and its shorter, hardier stature, to be easier to cultivate, and so it can be helpful to breed some of these characteristics into sativa strains.
- Crossbreeding can also be used to "mellow out" a sativa strain that tends to cause paranoia, or to decrease the tiredness caused by a certain type of indica.

CHAPTER 8

Plant secondary metabolites— terpenes/terpenoids

Those of you who are reading this and are medical herbalists will get entirely bored by my description of terpenes and terpenoids—because it is our bread and butter in many ways.

For everyone else, here is my favourite "cake analogy" in full.

Plants are like cakes—they have ingredients. It requires lots of different ingredients to make a good cake, and some cakes have more than others—the difference between a Madeira cake and a rich fruit cake for example. Plants are a bit like this too! These plant phytochemicals are called their primary or secondary metabolites. Many plants give off strong aromas and this is because they contain volatile oils. Everyone will instantly recognise the strong scent of lavender. Most people will also know that lavender is relaxing and soothing and it is used in bath oils, pillow sprays, and sleepy teas. A significant reason for this is the volatile oil contained within lavender, which is linalool. Interestingly, cannabis contains linalool too—some chemovars in greater and some in lesser quantities. So, different types of CBD products can be compared almost to different cakes—the Madeira cake, with a limited terpene profile in the plant—extremely basic. A cherry and sultana cake can be compared to a hybrid plant with a wider terpene profile, and a rich fruit cake compares favourably to an indica plant with its wide range of terpenes, flavonoids, and cannaflavins.

Cannabis, it transpires, contains an extremely wide array of terpenes (volatile oils) which is probably why it smells so pungently strong—possibly one of the most pungent plants you will ever encounter. That mixture of various volatile oils gives it its familiar aroma. Plant terpenoids are used extensively within aromatherapy and other complementary modalities for their aromatic qualities. Terpenes, monoterpenes, triterpenes, and sesquiterpenes, which are all under the "umbrella" term of "terpenes", have remarkable medicinal benefits in their own right!

There are more than 20,000 known terpenes in nature and over 100 are known to exist in cannabis and hemp.

Plants use terpenes to protect against herbivores and attract pollinators.

Terpenoids contribute to the scent of eucalyptus, the flavours of cinnamon, cloves, and ginger, the scent of lavender (known for its relaxing properties), and the scent and analgesic antibacterial effects of cloves.

Well-known terpenoids include limonene, linalool, myrcene, beta-caryophyllene, citral, menthol, camphor, and even salvinorin A which is found in the plant *Salvia divinorum*; the cannabinoids which are found in cannabis; plants such as *Ginkgo biloba* contain terpenoids called ginkgolide and bilobalide; and the curcuminoids found in turmeric and mustard seed.

The trichomes of the cannabis plant secrete the most diverse terpenoids of any plant in nature.

Common terpenes found in cannabis plants

What follows are just a few of the most common terpenes found in cannabis plants. As discussed, linalool, which smells

PLANT SECONDARY METABOLITES—TERPENES/TERPENOIDS 67

Common Terpenes in Cannabis

MYRCENE	LIMONENE	CARYOPHYLLENE	LINALOOL	PINENE
AROMA	**AROMA**	**AROMA**	**AROMA**	**AROMA**
Earthy	Citrus	Pepper	Floral	Pine
Cloves	Lemon	Wood	Sweet	Woody
Herbal	Orange	Spicy	Citrus	Mountain Air
FOUND IN	**FOUND IN**	**FOUND IN**	**FOUND IN**	**FOUND IN**
Hops	Citrus Fruits	Black Pepper	Lavender	Pine Needles
Fresh Mango	Peppermint	Cloves	Laurel	Parsley
Lemongrass	Juniper	Rosemary	Mints	Camphorweed
EFFECTS	**EFFECTS**	**EFFECTS**	**EFFECTS**	**EFFECTS**
Analgesic	Antidepressant	Analgesic	Analgesic	Anti-Inflammatory
Anti-Inflammatory	Antifungal	Anti-Inflammatory	Anti-Convulsant	Gastroprotective
Antipsychotic	Antimicrobial	Antidepressant	Anxiolytic	Energy Booster
Antispasmodic	Antispasmodic	Antiseptic	Sedative	Bronchodilator
Hypnotic	Anxiolytic	Protects Digestive	Antineoplastic	Anti-Bacterial
Muscle Relaxant	Gastroprotective	Tract	Antipsychotic	Memory Aid
Sedative	Immunostimulant	Cell Lining		

floral, sweet, and has that distinctive "lavender" smell, has a calming and relaxing effect. Medicinally it is anti-anxiety and sedating. Linalool is also found in rosewood.

Caryophyllene, which is found in black pepper and cloves, has a woody, spicy aroma, and can help with chronic pain and insomnia. An old wives' remedy is to chew a clove for toothache: this is because it is analgesic, antibacterial, and pain relieving—owing to its terpene profile. Pinene, as its name suggests, smells of pine trees, and enhances creativity, alertness, and can be euphoric. It is anti-inflammatory and can be of great help with asthma; it is also found in parsley, basil, and rosemary.

Limonene, as you can imagine, is found in citrus fruits and has a lemony smell—some cannabis plants are called "lemon haze" or "lemon kush" which is because they are rich in limonene and exude that citrusy smell. Its effects are stress relieving and mood elevating, good to use with anxiety and as an antidepressant. Interestingly limonene is also present in peppermint (*Mentha piperita*).

To aid the selection of potential terpenes and their medicinal benefits, I have created a "cheat sheet" which is easy to refer to.

Terpene	Also found in	Benefit	Aroma
Pinene	Parsley, basil, rosemary, pine needles	Anti-inflammatory, antibacterial, bronchodilator, aids memory	Pine, earth
Myrcene	Hops	Sedative, sleep aid, muscle relaxant	Flowers, pungent, earthy
Limonene	Citrus	Treats acid-reflux, anti-anxiety, antidepressant	Citrus, fresh spice
Terpinolene	Coriander	Analgesic, pain reducing, digestive aid	Pine, herbal, anise, lime
Linalool	Lavender, rosewood	Anaesthetic, anti-convulsive, analgesic, anti-anxiety	Flowers, lavender, citrus, fresh spice
Terpineol	Mugwort	Calming aid, antibacterial, antiviral, immune enhancing	Lilac, citrus, wood
Caryophyllene	Black pepper, cloves	Anti-inflammatory, analgesic, protects cell lining in digestive tract	Citrus, spice
Humulene	Hops, basil	Anti-inflammatory, relaxing	Robust, herbaceous, earthy

Individual terpenes — a closer look

Myrcene

- Myrcene, or beta-myrcene (β-myrcene), is a monoterpene that has a role as a plant metabolite, anti-inflammatory agent, anabolic agent, a fragrance, flavouring agent, and a volatile oil component, and is one of the most common terpenes produced by cannabis. Its aroma is most similar to cloves and has been 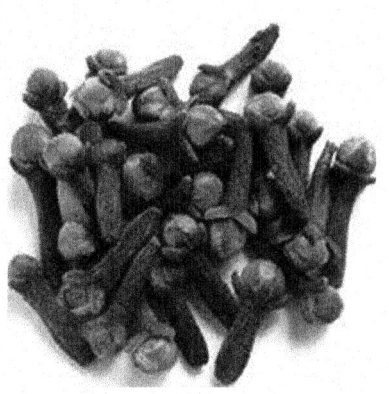 described as spicy, earthy, or musky. If a cannabis strain contains high levels of myrcene, it will be more relaxing and soporific. Plants rich in myrcene include laurel, parsley, thyme, hops, lemongrass, citrus fruits, bay leaves, and eucalyptus, among many others. Myrcene is probably the most researched of the terpenes within the cannabis plant and has huge therapeutic potential. Terpenes are generally secreted by the trichomes, the glandular heads of the cannabis plant.
- Myrcene has very particular medicinal properties and it has been shown that myrcene modifies the permeability of cell membranes thus lowering the resistance across the blood–brain barrier. This will allow chemicals to cross the blood–brain barrier more easily, including myrcene itself. When ingested within a cannabinoid, myrcene synergises with cannabinoids which in turn allows the effects to take place more quickly. It has also been shown to increase the maximum saturation level of the CB-1 receptor, which allows for a substantially greater psychoactive effect. Its sedative and

relaxing effects also make it ideal for the treatment of insomnia and pain.
- Myrcene is a strong analgesic and has anti-inflammatory, antibiotic and anti-antimutagenic properties. It can block the action of certain carcinogens. A 2014 study focused on the role of β-myrcene in preventing peptic ulcer disease. The study revealed that β-myrcene acts as an inhibitor of gastric and duodenal ulcers, suggesting it may be helpful in preventing peptic ulcer disease. A recent study carried out linked the myrcene content of a plant to its effect upon the human body. This research concluded that a higher level of myrcene is associated with the relaxing effects of indica strains, whilst a lower myrcene content would be more stimulating and thus confer the properties typical of a sativa plant.

Linalool

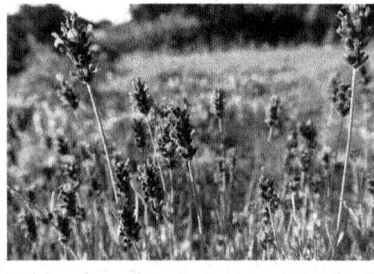

Linalool is a non-cyclic monoterpenoid which is commonly extracted from lavender, rose, basil, and orange blossom—its aroma is distinctly floral and reminiscent of lavender. A plant which has high levels of linalool will help to promote calmness and relaxation. Linalool has established sedative, antidepressant, anxiolytic, and immune potentiating effects and is found in significant quantities within the cannabis plant. Research has also indicated that linalool can have analgesic and anti-convulsant effects and is antinociceptive at high doses.

Historically, lavender has been used for centuries to aid sleep—lavender pillows, lavender water, and more recently "relaxing lavender plug-in air fresheners"; bubble baths, body rubs, and teas have been used for night-time relaxation. Linalool's anxiolytic properties make it a helpful ally particularly in modern times with anxiety and stress at record highs. Research has suggested linalool's usefulness in conditions such as post-traumatic stress or psychosis. There are even studies now suggesting that linalool may have immune boosting properties and anti-inflammatory properties particularly within the lung when inhaled, and thus it is becoming popular for conditions such as asthma and chronic obstructive pulmonary disorder (COPD).

Some studies have investigated the potential application of linalool in the treatment of dementia conditions owing to its purported ability to enhance cognitive and emotional function.

There has been research regarding the antifungal activity of linalool against conditions like conditions like thrush, which discovered that linalool inhibited and suppressed certain pathways indicating it could have therapeutic potential in the treatment of candidiasis because of the way it interferes with the morphological switch and biofilm formation of candida albicans.

A study published in 2016 found that linalool reversed neuropathological and behavioural impairments in mice with Alzheimer's disease. The linalool improved learning and spatial memory and the subjects exhibited a significant reduction of pro-inflammatory markers, indicating that linalool could restore cognitive and emotional functions via an anti-inflammatory effect. It was felt that there should be further research into using linalool as a potential treatment for Alzheimer's.

Several studies have looked at the inhalation of linalool and its effect on airway inflammation and have concluded that oral administration of linalool significantly inhibited eosinophil numbers, and that it had a preventative effect upon inflammatory cells and mucus hypersecretion in lung tissues. One study looked at the inhibition of cigarette smoke harm and indicated that linalool could block carcinogenesis and could be helpful in reducing the harm caused by inhaling cigarette smoke.

Linalool is frequently used in a wide variety of bath and body products and is often listed under ingredients as not only linalool but linalyl alcohol, linaloyl oxide, p-linalool, and allo-ocimenol. The vapours of linalool have shown significant effects as an insecticide against fruit flies, fleas, and cockroaches.

Linalool is prolific and has been isolated in hundreds of different plants. It can be found within the Lamiaceae (mint) family which includes many scented herbs and the Lauraceae (laurel) families as well as the Rutaceae plant family (citrus plants amongst others). This therefore includes mint, cinnamon, rosewood, and many other aromatic herbs. A variety of tropical plants as well as birch trees have also been found to contain linalool. Linalool is a crucial antecedent in vitamin E formation.

Limonene

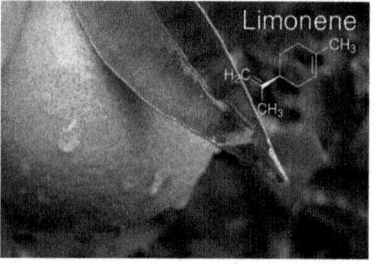

- Limonene is a monocyclic monoterpenoid and is one of the most common terpenes found in nature. It is found in the rind of citrus fruits, particularly orange peel, the oil content of which is made up of approximately 97% limonene. It is also one of two major compounds formed from pinene. As its name suggests it has a citrus-like aroma, reminiscent of lemons, limes, and oranges and is additionally found in the rinds of these and other citrus fruits such as grapefruit. Limonene is also found in other herbs and plants such as rosemary, juniper, peppermint, and some pine needle oil, as well as the seeds of caraway and dill.
- Plants produce secondary metabolites to aid their own growth and survival and limonene is a natural insecticide and thus can deter predators.

- Interestingly, as initially limonene was not considered for "health benefits" and it is a by-product of the world's huge consumption of orange juice, until around thirty years ago it was sold to cleaning companies for use in household products, detergents, shampoos, lotions, perfumes, soaps, and many more. Used also as a flavouring in the food industry and because it is completely biodegradable and non-toxic, this has led to its popularity by companies seeking to create environmentally friendly products. It is considered to have very low toxicity; however, it has been noted that some extremely sensitive people are allergic to some terpenes and limonene and linalool have such very strong fragrances that these seem to be the main culprits in those scenarios.
- As an essential oil, limonene is considered calming, mood elevating, and to have many other therapeutic properties.
- Limonene is a precursor and component of mint and the refreshing taste of mint is owing to its limonene content.
- Research shows that limonene rapidly enters the bloodstream as it is highly absorbed by inhalation. It allows other terpenes to be absorbed through pores of the skin and is thus often used in skin cream products. It has also been documented that limonene can suppress fungal and bacterial growth making it an ideal product for inclusion in antifungal products for conditions such as tinea pedis. It is believed to be a beneficial anti-cancer protectant and there are current trials underway examining its benefits in the treatment of breast cancers. Limonene has also shown another benefit in helping to promote weight reduction.

Caryophyllene

Beta-caryophyllene is a natural bicyclic sesquiterpene that is a constituent of a great variety of essential oils, in particular in *Syzygium aromaticum* (cloves) but is also found in cannabis, black pepper, cinnamon leaves, allspice, fig, pot marjoram, and roman chamomile, as well as in lavender, albeit in minor quantities. The aroma of caryophyllene is woody, spicy, and peppery and it is unique in that it may not only be described as a terpene but also as a

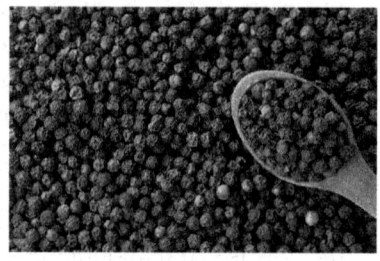

cannabinoid. This is because it is the only terpene known to interact with the endocannabinoid system (CB-2). It selectively activates CB-2 receptors and is a functional CB-2 agonist and yet these characteristics were only discovered as recently as 2008 by a team of German researchers. It was further discovered that caryophyllene was a functional non-psychoactive CB-2 receptor ligand in foodstuffs and is a macrocyclic anti-inflammatory. Its ability to fight inflammation and aid in the recovery from substance addiction holds further promise that this important terpene may be medicinally extraordinarily valuable in the future.

- A study by Varga et al. published in 2018 by the *British Journal of Pharmacology* entitled "Beta-Caryophyllene Protects against Alcoholic Steatohepatitis by Attenuating Inflammation", concluded that given its safety in humans, β-caryophyllene had a "high translational potential in treating or preventing hepatic injury associated with oxidative stress, inflammation and steatosis".
- In 2014, a research paper entitled "β-caryophyllene, a CB-2 receptor agonist produces multiple behavioural changes relevant to anxiety and depression in mice" was published and concluded that BCP displayed anti-anxiety effects, was antidepressant, suggested that CB-2 receptors may be targeted in the treatment of anxiety and depression, and suggested that "the possibility that beta-caryophyllene may ameliorate the symptoms of mood disorders offers exciting prospects for future studies".

- A paper published in October 2013 by Perry Fine and Mark Rosenfeld looked at specific roles of endocannabinoids that act as ligands at endogenous cannabinoid receptors within the central nervous system and found that these did exert an influence on nociception. They found that oral administration of cannabidiol and beta caryophyllene appeared to show extraordinary promise in the treatment of chronic pain, attenuated by the low adverse effects and high safety profiles of these substances.
- A study published in 2012 suggested that β-caryophyllene, via its CB-2 receptor-dependent pathway could be of outstanding value as a therapeutic to prevent nephrotoxicity (kidney poisoning) which was a result of chemotherapy drugs such as cisplatin. They discovered that β-caryophyllene diminishes cisplatin-induced kidney inflammation, oxidative stress, and injury, and confirmed that the protective effect of β-caryophyllene is mediated via the CB-2 receptors.
- A series of studies between 2011 and 2015 by Liju et al. evaluated the chemical composition of essential oils extracted from *Curcuma longa* (turmeric) and *Zingiber officinalis* (ginger) of which caryophyllene is a main constituent. They discovered its antioxidant, anti-inflammatory, and antinociceptive (pain-relieving) properties. This suggests strongly that strains high in caryophyllene could be extremely useful in treating a wide variety of conditions such as arthritis, neuropathic pain, and muscular aches and pains such as fibromyalgia.

Pinene

- Pinene is a bicyclic monoterpenoid. Aromatically resembling pine or fir, pinene has two structural isomers namely: α-pinene and β-pinene. Both are found in many species of coniferous trees as well as in essential oil of rosemary (*Rosmarinus officinalis*). Both types of pinene are the major components of pine resin; however, α-pinene is one of the most prolific terpenoids found in nature. Even some citrus fruits contain α-pinene and together the two 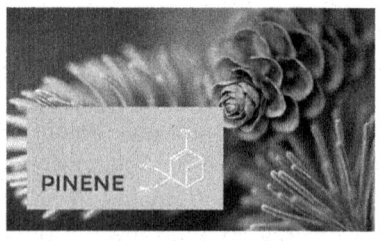 isomers make up the main component in wood turpentine. Pinene is one of the most important monoterpenes as it is significant to the physiology of both plants and animals. Pinene has a tendency to react with many other chemicals and metabolites and is a precursor to other terpenes such as limonene and other composites.

- Medicinally, pinene has anti-inflammatory, expectorant, broncho-dilating, and local antiseptic properties, making it of immense value. When it is isolated α-pinene has demonstrated anti-cancer activity and has historically been used for this purpose within traditional Chinese medicine for quite some time. Studies have indicated that the effects of THC may be ameliorated if there is a significant amount of pinene present.
- Rosemary for remembrance is a well-known adage, and this is owing to its pinene content. In studies pinene has demonstrated the ability to help prevent short-term memory loss, enhance mental alertness, and with its bronchodilatory properties can improve airflow to the respiratory system. This could be of great benefit to asthma and chronic obstructive pulmonary disorder (COPD) sufferers as well as those with other pulmonary conditions.
- Studies have shown that pinene has tumour-shrinking properties which could be of great value in cancer cases.

So how does pinene work?

- It is claimed that pinene has an effect on the permeability of cell membranes particularly the blood–brain barrier,

increasing transport of cannabinoids into the brain, and thus acting upon neurotransmitters and thereby enhancing short-term memory, although there is a lack of hard data to confirm this theory.
- Nevertheless, it appears that the use of cannabis products rich in pinene amongst other terpenoids often results in a high level of alertness and clarity of mind.
- Alpha-pinene is found in large quantities in tea tree (*Melaleuca*) and was used in aboriginal medicine to treat open wounds and prevent infections. In modern times tea tree is used prolifically in mouthwash, handwash, cough lozenges, chest ointments, hand sanitisers, and many other products as an antibacterial agent.
- Recent studies have shown that a-pinene exhibits anti-inflammatory effects in human chondrocytes—thereby exhibiting potential anti-osteoarthritic activity. Further studies should be carried out for the promising activity as an anti-osteoarthritic.

Humulene

Humulene is a sesquiterpene of hops (*Humulus lupulus*), with a familiar "hoppy" aroma, however it is additionally found in other plants such as sage, ginseng, Vietnamese coriander, and cannabis. It is a ring-opened isomer 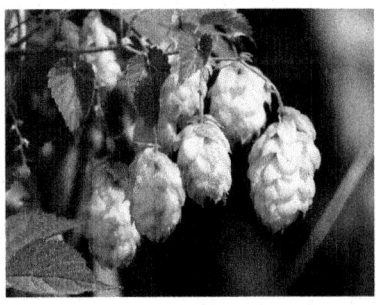 of β-caryophyllene and is also known as α-humulene and α-caryophyllene. It is lacking in CB-2 activity but in studies has shown to be as anti-inflammatory as dexamethasone in an animal model. The distinctive aroma of hops in beer is caused by humulene. It possesses both topical and systemic anti-inflammatory properties as well as inducing relaxation and sleep.

- A 2006 study examined the sedating effects of *Humulus lupulus* (hops) CO2 extracts, and discovered that it reduced spontaneous locomotor activity and increased sleeping time, confirming a central sedating effect—this could show promise with conditions such as Parkinson's. As an aside to this, I have had a patient with benign essential tremor, who always found that after a beer, the tremor subsided, and he was able to function more normally.
- A study in 2008 looked at the preventative and therapeutic potential of a-humulene in allergic inflammation in the airways and found that it exhibited marked anti-inflammatory properties on airways' allergic inflammation via a reduction of inflammatory mediators.
- Studies have suggested that humulene may be anti-tumour, but is also found to be antibacterial, anti-inflammatory, and appetite suppressing. In a study in 2019 a-humulene was found to have significant anti hepatocellular carcinoma activity both in vitro and in vivo. The researchers found that humulene was cytotoxic to the cancer cells and induced their apoptosis, although showing minimal cytotoxicity to normal hepatocytes. The subjects were also observed to lose weight.
- It has been used for many years in traditional Chinese medicine. When blended with β-caryophyllene it has been used as a significant remedy for inflammation. It aids in weight loss by acting as an appetite suppressant.

Terpinolene

Terpinolene is a monoterpene and is found in sage, rosemary, apple, tea tree, cumin, and nutmeg. Its strongly aromatic features mean it is used prolifically in soaps, perfumes, lotions, and particular insect repellents. It has a piney or woody aroma with a slight herbal or floral undertone. Its flavour resembles citrus fruits.

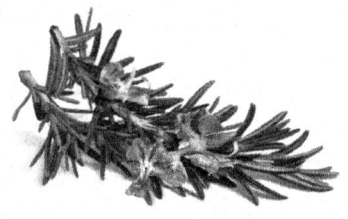

Within cannabis terpinolene is thought to have a mildly sedative effect as well as being anxiolytic, balancing out the energetic qualities of a sativa plant. It is generally only found in sativa dominant chemovars. Terpinolene appears to have no analgesic or anti-inflammatory properties in the way that many other terpenes do and is not as prevalent within the plant as other terpenes such as limonene or myrcene. It does, however, display some antiseptic properties.

Terpinolene has been found to be a central nervous system depressant when used to induce drowsiness or sleep or to reduce psychological excitement or anxiety. Further, terpinolene was found to markedly reduce the protein expression of AKT1 in K562 cells and inhibited cell proliferation involved in a variety of human cancers.

Camphene

Camphene, a plant-derived monoterpene, emits pungent odours of damp woodlands and fir needles. It is virtually insoluble in water, but highly soluble in organic solvents. It is a minor constituent of a variety of essential oils including turpentine, cypress oil, camphor,

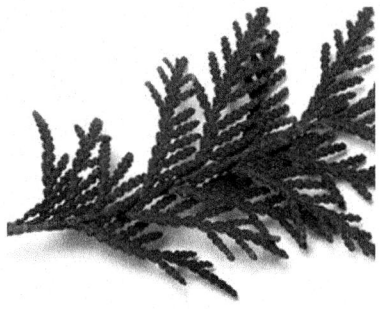

citronella, neroli, and valerian. It is used in fragrances and some foodstuffs as an aromatic.

A study in 2011 discovered that camphene reduced plasma cholesterol and triglycerides in hyperlipidaemic rats. Bearing in mind the almost epidemic proportions of statin prescription, which have been shown to cause intestinal issues, liver damage, and muscular inflammation, the potential for camphene to be used as an alternative to pharmaceutical lipid-lowering agents holds some promise.

Phellandrene

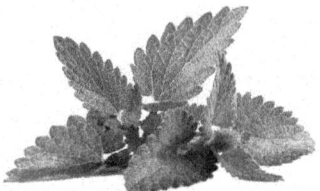

Alpha phellandrene was named after *Eucalyptus phellandra* (now termed *Eucalyptus radiata*) from which it was originally isolated. Its aroma is described as peppermint with a hint of citrus and it is believed to have an array of medicinal values. It has been used in traditional Chinese medicine to treat digestive disorders and is also one of the main compounds in turmeric leaf oil which has antifungal properties.

However, phellandrene is found only in such tiny quantities that research has been limited and it is believed that despite its ease of identification in the laboratory setting it is not available in large enough quantities to be of significant medicinal value.

As stated, phellandrene was first found in eucalyptus oil. However, it wasn't until the mid-1900s that science had moved forward enough that it could be isolated, and the discovery was made that phellandrene from eucalyptus oil contained two isomers of phellandrene (more often than not alluded to as α-phellandrene and β-phellandrene), and on oxidation with potassium permanganate gave distinct acids which proved that the acids had been acquired from two different isomeric phellandrenes. Prior to this time, phellandrene was taken to be pinene or limonene. Currently a wide variety of essential oils are known that contain phellandrene. However, it is an unreliable terpene as there are only some species in which it can be detected, especially the eucalypts and that only at certain times of the year.

Phellandrene is found in herbs such as cinnamon, garlic, dill, ginger, and parsley. Lavender produces β-phellandrene as a constituent of its essential oil. Certain aromas of essential oils are entirely a consequence of the constituent phellandrene, in particular pepper, dill, and ginger essential oils. Phellandrene absorbs trans-dermally particularly well and thus is popularly used in perfume and skincare manufacture. Apparently, there is also some scant use of this product as a flavouring in certain food products.

Various studies have been carried out looking at phellandrene's anti-inflammatory and wound healing actions and have found a significant role for phellandrene as an anti-inflammatory agent.

Carene

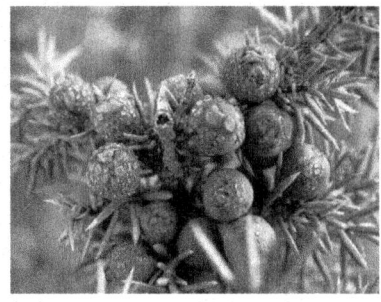

Delta-3-carene is a bicyclic monoterpene with a sweet citrusy odour. It can be found in a wide variety of essential oils, in particular juniper berry oil, cypress oil, and fir needle essential oil. Studies have learnt that delta-3-carene can depress the central nervous system and has anhydrous properties which gives it potential for clinical use to improve conditions such as hyperhidrosis

Delta-3-carene has a low toxicity although inhalation could cause irritation. It is also naturally occurring in pine extract, bell pepper, basil, grapefruit, orange, and citrus peel oils. Carene is a significant component of turpentine and is also used as a flavouring in certain products.

Studies have indicated that carene has been implicated in assisting with differentiation and stimulation of calcium production in bone cells. It has also been found to have mosquito repellent properties.

Terpineol

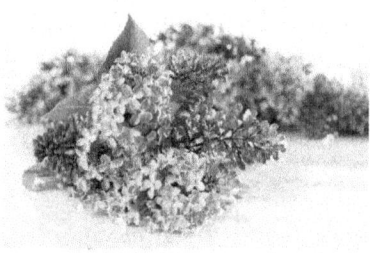

α-terpineol, terpinen-4-ol, and 4-terpineol are three closely related monoterpenoids. The aroma of terpineol has been compared to lilacs and flower blossoms and is a frequently used ingredient in perfumes, cosmetics, and flavourings. It is one of the most abundant aromas in lapsang souchong tea, which originates from the pine smoke used to dry the tea. It is often found in certain cannabis varieties which simultaneously have higher pinene levels and the strong aroma of the pinene overshadows the terpineol making it indistinguishable.

Terpineol, specifically α-terpineol, is known to have calming, relaxing effects. It also exhibits antibiotic, AChE inhibitor, antioxidant and antimalarial properties. There has been some research into its antidiarrhoeal activity by its inhibition of vagal parasympathetic pathways.

Pulegone

Pulegone, a monocyclic monoterpenoid, is a minor component of cannabis. Higher concentrations of pulegone are found in rosemary. Rosemary breaks down acetylcholine in the brain, allowing nerve cells to communicate more effectively with one another.

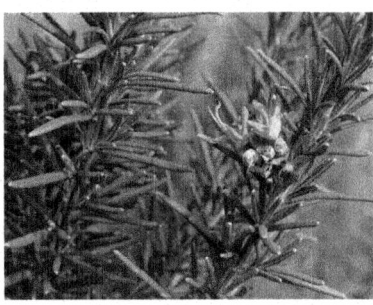

Studies indicate that more than 85% of pulegone occurs in the pennyroyal plant but is also found in smaller quantities in the leaves and flowers of the Lamiaceae (mint) family. Interestingly it is also present in the leaves of *Barosma betulina* (buchu) which may explain buchu's blackcurrant menthol flavour.

Within plants that contain large percentages of pulegone, the herbal properties are vast and it contributes to their medicinal benefits in cases such as dyspepsia, menstrual cramps, endometriosis pain, oligomenorrhoea, secondary amenorrhoea, and in some of the mint family plants it contributes to diuretic, common cold relief, headache relief, vomiting, spasms, and has soothing propensity for the symptoms of inflammatory bowel syndrome or IBS.

Studies have been performed to look at the benefits of pulegone for its potential as an antioxidant, antimicrobial, and insect repellent among many other uses.

An ethnopharmacology study indicates pulegone may have significant sedative and fever-reducing properties.

Sabinene

Sabinene is a bicyclic monoterpene which has an aroma that might remind some of Christmas as it has a pine, orange, and spicy or woody scent. It appears in a large variety of plants, among which are black pepper and nutmeg—in fact it gives black pepper its spicy and hot nature. It is used to add flavour to carrots and the discernible earthy green flavour of carrot is directly attributable to sabinene. It is believed to have anti-inflammatory and antibacterial properties.

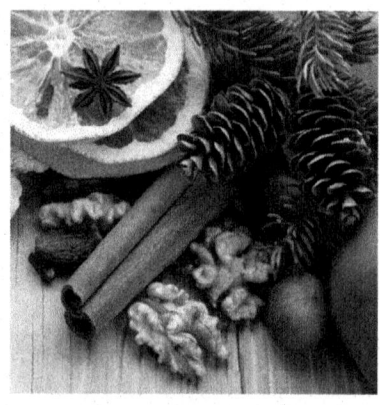

Results of a 2013 study by Valente et al. suggest that sabinene (in combination with myrcene) should be explored further as a natural source of new antioxidant and anti-inflammatory drugs for the development of food supplements, nutraceuticals, or plant-based medicines.

Sabinene is present in tea tree oil and it is thought that this adds to the antibacterial and antifungal properties of the oil.

Geraniol

Geraniol is a monoterpenoid and an alcohol. As a compound it has a fragrance that is strongly reminiscent of roses. This has made geraniol an extremely popular choice for many toiletries, perfumes, and bath products.

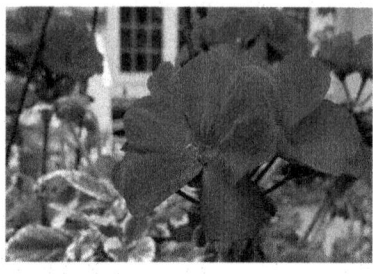

It is found in roses, palmarosa, and citronella. This makes geraniol-based products a highly effective mosquito repellent. Some research shows that geraniol shows promise in the treatment of neuropathy.

Geraniol is an alcohol-based terpene and thus is insoluble in water. It is occasionally also used in food product flavouring.

CHAPTER 9

Flavonoids and cannaflavins

Often overlooked are the flavonoids, most people concentrating more on the cannabinoids THC and CBD and then the terpenes; however, flavonoids are also a very important component of cannabis as a medicinal herb. Flavonoids can be found in most plants, fruits, and vegetables and give fruits, vegetables, and plants a yellow, orange, or red colour. They are all antioxidant which has a beneficial effect on the heart and circulation, enhancing resilience to stress and strengthening and healing blood vessels. Flavonoids are anti-inflammatory, can be hepatoprotective, anti-tumour, antiviral and hypotensive. Herbs rich in flavonoids can be cardioprotective and help to treat vascular problems as well as helping to protect connective tissue.

There are thought to be around 6000 different flavonoids—these are separated into six individual categories.

Anthoxanthins
These flavonoids are water soluble and produce pigments that are white or yellow. Examples of anthoxanthin flavonoids include quercetin, galangin, and luteolin.

Flavanones
Believed to play a critical role in plant cell growth, this category of flavonoid is aromatic and colourless. It is commonly found in tomatoes, mint, and citrus. Some flavonoids in this category include naringin, butin, and hesperetin.

Flavanols
Also colourless, flavanols play a vital role in inhibiting plant cell growth. Examples of this flavonoid include orientin, taxifolin, and aromadendrin.

Flavans
Flavans create bitter and acidic flavours in foods. They are most commonly found in the tannins of unripe fruits and vegetables, as well as wine, tea, and cocoa. Some of the flavonoids that belong to this group include catechins, theaflavin, and thearubigin.

Anthocyanidins
This group of flavonoids is responsible for the vivid blue, red, and purple pigmentations found in common foods like radishes, sweet potatoes, berries, and even some tomato varieties. Examples of anthocyanidin flavonoids include capensinidin, hirsutidin, and cyanidin.

And most interestingly of all ...

Cannaflavins
These flavonoids only exist in cannabis. There are only three cannaflavins: they have been rather mundanely named cannaflavin A, cannaflavin B, and cannaflavin C. Of these the one with the most research is cannaflavin A.

Cannaflavins are believed to work in conjunction with other flavonoids to give distinctive aromas, tastes, and pigmentations to cannabis strains.

The many health benefits of flavonoids

Scientists believe there are roughly twenty flavonoids present in cannabis, and many share the same therapeutic properties. Here is a look at some of the most common flavonoids and their benefits:

Aromadendrin
Benefits: anti-inflammatory and cancer-fighting properties

Butin
Benefits: reduces oxidative stress-related cell dysfunction

Cannaflavin A
Benefits: anti-inflammatory, antifungal, antioxidant, and cancer-fighting properties

Cannaflavin B and cannaflavin C
Benefits: anti-inflammatory, antifungal, antioxidant, and cancer-fighting properties

Catechins
Benefits: anti-inflammatory, antioxidant, and helps lower cholesterol

Galangin
Benefits: antioxidative, immunoprotective, cardioprotective properties and tumour-fighting properties

Hesperetin
Benefits: improves blood vessel conditions, anti-carcinogenic, antioxidant, and anti-inflammatory

Isovitexin
Benefits: antioxidant, anti-cancer, anti-inflammatory, anti-hyperalgesic, and neuroprotective effects

Luteolin
Benefits: antioxidative, tumour-fighting, and anti-inflammatory properties

Naringin
Benefits: antioxidant, anti-carcinogenic, and helps lower cholesterol

Orientin
Benefits: antioxidant, antiviral, antibacterial, anti-inflammatory, cardioprotective, and neuroprotective

Quercetin
Benefits: pain relief, reduces inflammation, cardioprotective properties, cancer-fighting properties, immunoprotective, and eases skin irritation when used topically

Taxifolin
Benefits: supports cardiovascular health, improves cognitive function, and immunoprotective

Vitexin
Benefits: antioxidant, anti-cancer, anti-inflammatory, anti-hyperalgesic, and neuroprotective effects

Generally speaking, research is showing that flavonoids are beneficial for treating haemorrhoids, boosting the immune system, reducing the risk of stroke, and fighting cancer.

Flavonoids and cancer

Cancer is a condition that involves abnormal cell growth which can become invasive and spread to various organs or body parts and it is obviously a significant public health concern worldwide. Cancer research and the search for a cure or amelioration of malignancy is a constant battle in many developed countries. Many plant-derived pharmaceutical anti-cancer agents are in clinical use worldwide such as vincristine, vinblastine, taxol, topotecan, irinotecan, and etoposide, among many others. Several other promising plant-derived anti-cancer agents are becoming increasingly popular such as salvestrols, flavopirodol, roscovitine, and betulinic acid. The plant derivatives of these products are dominant in polyphenols and flavonoids.

Studies have considered that a major cause of cancer(s) is an excess of free radicals—which creates a mutation in otherwise healthy cells as time goes on. Such cells then distort and create tumours, spreading or metastasising throughout the body.

Scientists believe that flavonoids could not only aid the prevention of the formation of cancer cells by their free radical stabilisation qualities, but it seems they also have antiproliferative actions, which means the spread of cancer could be halted entirely. It is also mooted that these flavonoids could increase the rate of cell apoptosis (cell death).

Numerous studies have been carried out and are constantly ongoing regarding the use of flavonoids in conditions such as oral, breast, prostate, lung, and colon cancers as well as leukaemia.

There has been a positive correlation between lower levels of cancers and other health issues in communities where flavonoid consumption is high. It has been noted that death from cancer is less common in countries where high levels of flavonoids are consumed as part of a typical diet. Studies have shown, for example, with the Mediterranean diet or the Okinawa diet, people suffer far less significant health issues and less occurrence of cancer. The Okinawa diet is based around a small series of islands in Japan, of which the largest is Okinawa. The local population have a diet that is extraordinarily rich in brightly coloured vegetables, notably the purple sweet potato—packed full of flavonoids. The longevity of Okinawa's inhabitants is legendary with the largest number of centenarians in the world. This is largely ascribed to the diet which is rich in turmeric, seaweed, and fish as well as colourful vegetables, and low in sugars and refined foods. Since 2000, the diet in Okinawa has changed slightly with the younger population keen to try some of the "modern" foods rather than sticking to the historical diet. It seems that this has caused the longevity of islanders to drop slightly.

Flavonoids and cannabis

Cannabinoids and terpenes are the "pop stars" of the cannabis plant and flavonoids have been barely considered; however, flavonoids are in fact vastly more copious in cannabis plants than their famous cousins.

At least two dozen different flavonoids have thus far been found in the cannabis plant, many of which are of the flavanol and flavanone variety. Flavonoids such as kaempferol which is found in tea, broccoli, cabbage, kale, beans, endive, leeks, tomatoes, strawberries, and grapes, and in herbal medicines such as *Ginkgo biloba*, tilia, equisetum, moringa, and propolis; also in quercetin which is found in red wine (that's why it's good for you!), onions, green tea, apples, berries, *Ginkgo biloba*, and St John's wort amongst others. These are both well-researched antioxidant flavonoids with a wide variety of health benefits.

Cannabis also contains its very own group of flavonoids—considered to have highly effective anti-inflammatory actions, as previously mentioned; these are cannaflavin A, cannaflavin B, and cannaflavin C.

Other flavonoids discovered in the cannabis plant include apigenin—which is also found in large quantities in both Roman chamomile (*Chamaemelum nobile*) and German chamomile (*Matricaria recutita*) as well as in many other herbs and plants such as brahmi (*Bacopa monnieri*). Apigenin has been found to induce auto phagocytosis (cell destruction) in leukaemia cells and it may be considered both a metabolite and an antineoplastic agent. It has also shown significant positive results as a skin cancer chemoprotective agent.

A further flavonoid found prolifically within cannabis is luteolin, which is also found in broccoli, celery, green pepper, and thyme (*Thymus vulgaris*). Research has discovered it is antioxidant, anti-inflammatory and possesses beneficial neuroprotective effects as well as being chemoprotective and immunomodulatory.

The other types of flavonoids found in cannabis plants are anthocyanins which are the secondary metabolites that impart vibrant colours to plants and are particularly prominent in strains which are purple.

Flavonoids not only affect the colour of the cannabis plant, but also its aroma and flavour, as well as imparting a wide variety of health benefits. Aroma and flavour are, however, also partially due to the terpene content of the plant.

Terpenes and cannabinoids are predominantly found in the trichomes that cover cannabis buds and flowers whereas flavonoids are present throughout the entire plant, including stems, leaves, and seeds which are often discarded and considered inconsequential. However, this is incorrect; it transpires these "inconsequential" parts may have additional health benefits to offer, so when looking for oil, "whole-plant extract" is something to aim for.

The "entourage effect"

An entourage is a group of people who support one important person, and because of the way that the cannabinoids, terpenes, flavonoids, and other phytochemical ingredients appear to work synergistically within the cannabis plant to provide a greater and more beneficial effect, the term "entourage effect" came into being. It was first coined by Israeli scientist Raphael Mechoulam. As medical herbalists we are very aware of the fact that the entire plant contains benefits more than its individual phytochemicals—take out one ingredient and side effects occur which is why isolated compounds or synthesised isolates are not as effective as a whole plant medicine. Taking CBD or THC or CBN in complete isolation would not be as effective as taking a whole-plant extract. This is confirmed in the way that the negative effects of THC are balanced out by CBD, for example.

However, cannabinoids aside, the terpenes and flavonoids within the plant also have an important role to play. Current thinking is that flavonoids enhance the bioavailability of other cannabis compounds, influencing how they are transported around the body and altering how they bind with receptors. There is also a consideration that flavonoids influence cytochrome P-450, the enzymatic pathway in the liver involved in the metabolism of all drugs, medicines, certain foodstuffs, and obviously cannabis.

Since the phrase "the entourage effect" came into being, people have focused specifically on this—promoting the effect as a beneficial manifestation which modulates the therapeutic effects of cannabis. This expression has become so "hyped up" and promoted by various manufacturers and suppliers of CBD products that it has possibly lost its original meaning. To me, it simply means that the product is a broad-spectrum product made from whole-plant matter, rather than an isolate. The added bonus of all those flavonoids, terpenes, and cannaflavins enhances the medicinal properties of cannabidiol (CBD) as well as the other cannabinoids and phytochemicals.

CHAPTER 10

Herbs that work synergistically with cannabis

As medical herbalists we have a huge pharmacopeia of herbs to choose from, and we often use these in combination with each other because they work so well synergistically. A very typical example here would be turmeric, which is usually combined with a pepper of some description (which could be black pepper, ginger, or the Ayurvedic combination trikatu) because the addition of the pepper enhances the bioavailability of the turmeric. To a herbalist, using one herb as a "simple" or in isolation is often useful, but a lot of herbalists have told me that they find the use of cannabis as a panacea for all ills to be far too reductionist. Invariably herbalists like to select different herbs to work for different conditions pertinent and unique to each patient.

With regard to herbal synergy, however, there are some that have been found to have a particular affinity and interaction with cannabis. Some internet research has come up with lots of wonderful recipes for balms, lotions, and potions that include herbal medicines we know and love with the addition of some CBD. There are now even cookbooks and recipe books dedicated to creating CBD oil foodstuffs, sweets, gummies, chocolates, cakes, brownies (well there would have to be brownies of course), salads, and many more.

Cannabis and lavender

The mint family (Lamiaceae) produces many herbs that seem to work particularly well when combined with cannabis. Lavender (*Lavandula* spp) is just one. Lavender on its own is carminative, antispasmodic, analgesic, antioxidant, and antidepressant—amongst its many other qualities. Lavender essential oil makes a fabulous burn aid—it can heal burned skin very quickly and every kitchen should keep a bottle of lavender essential oil near the cooker. Lavender is also calming! You can buy lavender room sprays, plug-ins, and even lavender flavoured chews for dogs to calm them down. In herbal medicine lavender is used to aid and relieve digestion and colic, for anxiety, headaches, migraines, to lift the spirits, for colds, coughs, and the flu; it's decongestant and can relieve asthma; the rosmarinic acid in it has antioxidant and anti-inflammatory actions, and externally it's amazing for burns. In practice I have found lavender essential oil a wonderful aid for migraines when used topically.

Cannabis and lavender both have abundant quantities of the terpene linalool—as discussed in the previous chapter, linalool has a wide variety of applications but combined with cannabis its anti-inflammatory and pain-relieving properties are enhanced dramatically. Topically this has many applications for anti-inflammatory creams and balms, massage oils and so forth, but could also be ingested in the form of lavender cannabis chocolate—with added amazing anandamide in the cacao, or brownies, cakes, biscuits, and so forth.

Cannabis and rosemary

Rosemary (*Rosmarinus off.*) as well as cannabis and black pepper all contain beta-caryophyllene (abbreviated to BCP). BCP interacts with cannabinoid receptors and enhances the bioavailability of products through the enzymatic pathway

CYP450 and its family of enzymes. In my stores I have been selling a turmeric, frankincense. and pepper capsule for years—the BCP in the pepper enhances bioavailability of the turmeric and frankincense, and it is now pretty much common knowledge with the general public that they have to take their turmeric with some pepper. Some CBD manufacturers are adding piperine or pepper into cannabis products for the same reason. Whole-plant extract should contain some BCP but interestingly upon ingestion BCP binds itself to cannabinoid receptor 2 (CB-2) in the body, which enhances the immunological and inflammatory responses, helping to regulate them.

As discussed in the section on β-caryophyllene this can relieve symptoms of depression and anxiety. "Rosemary for remembrance" is something one often hears; well, this is because the rosemary also contains the terpene pinene which is also found in cannabis, and there is scientific research indicating it can help enhance memory.

Cannabis and holy basil

Holy basil (*Ocimum sanctum*), known in Ayurvedic medicine as tulsi, is an extremely sacred plant in India. It has been used for at least the last 5000 years medicinally, and as it contains β-caryophyllene in high quantities as well as cinnamic acid (also found in cinnamon) its health benefits are diverse. Holy basis is used for mentally uplifting and cleansing and purifying the atmosphere. Its essential oils contain linalool, eugenol, and camphor. It can be used topically for pain and makes a great addition to a CBD salve or cream.

In combination with CBD, research has shown that holy basil can enhance stress-reduction and is anxiolytic; this is owing to the fact that it has been found to reduce cortisol in clinical trials. Several studies have examined the anti-inflammatory action of holy basil. It contains phytochemicals which inhibit the production of inflammatory prostaglandins, enhancing its pain-relieving and anti-inflammatory effects.

Cannabis and echinacea

Echinacea, which is commonly used to boost the immune system in those suffering from coughs and colds, also contains cannabis like phytochemicals which interact with the endocannabinoid system. The alkamides, also known as alkylamides, within echinacea, called N-acylethanolamines (NAEs), interact with enzymes that break down endocannabinoids within the body and also interact with the CB-2 receptor. These alkamides are known as "cannabimimetic" because these compounds are so similar to cannabis. Alkamides are lipophilic constituents predominantly found in the roots of *Echinacea angustifolia* and also *Echinacea purpurea*. Because of their affinity to CB-2 receptors, they are also considered cannabis ligands. Studies suggest that this is what makes echinacea such an outstanding immunomodulator.

Cannabis and black cohosh

Studies have shown that women undergoing premature menopause are low in endocannabinoid levels; and thus increasing these, or activating the cannabinoid receptors in these women, may help with perimenopausal and menopausal symptoms. As previously discussed, cannabis can help with many of the side effects of the menopause such as mood swings, sleep issues, hot flushes, and bone density. Black cohosh (*Cimicifuga racemosa* or *Actea racemosa*) contains phytoestrogens, and as a result it is often used to alleviate symptoms of menopause. Synergistically the two herbs together (cannabis and black cohosh) could certainly be useful in the managing of peri-menopausal, menopausal, and postmenopausal symptoms.

Cannabis and ashwagandha

Withania somnifera, commonly known as ashwagandha, is an Indian Ayurvedic herb used for *rasayana*, which is the practice of replenishment of energy and rejuvenation of the body. It is one of the most fundamental healing plants in the Ayurvedic *Materia Medica* and is also known as "Indian ginseng" due to its rejuvenating properties. Apparently, the aroma of the root of the ashwagandha plant resembles horse sweat and it transpires that the Sanskrit word "ashwagandha" literally translates as "smell of the horse". In ancient tradition the herb was believed to impart the strength and vitality of a stallion to its user. It now transpires that ancient traditions are sometimes remarkably close to the truth. Modern studies have confirmed that ashwagandha is a booster of testosterone and increased sperm count and motility in a study of seventy-five infertile men. It is believed to enhance the sexual health of women just as successfully.

With regard to post-traumatic stress disorder (PTSD), a study concluded that *Withania somnifera* could prevent memory impairment resulting from this condition. It was posited that this effect was through preserving changes in antioxidant mechanisms in the hippocampus of the brain. A further contemporary study, completed in 2019, examined the amelioration of neurodegeneration and cognitive impairments associated with system inflammation and considered that ashwagandha was a promising natural therapeutic in this regard.

An extensive study completed in August of 2019 closely examined the evidence for the therapeutic application of *Withania somnifera* in cancer cases and concluded that there is significant potential for it to be utilised in such cases.

Withania somnifera is an adaptogenic herb that is thought to be relatively safe, although to be employed with care or avoided during pregnancy and breastfeeding and also for those people on immunosuppressant medication. However, in modern use, *Withania* is sold in supplementation form to support and alleviate such conditions as stress and anxiety, blood sugar control, immune response, fertility, testosterone levels, muscle development, and memory enhancement.

As antidepressant studies have shown there has been significant benefit in the reduction of severe depression. Withania also has antioxidant properties akin to CBD, improving cell-mediated immunity. High daily doses of ashwagandha root resulted in increased muscle mass, size, and strength in men who participated in a study after only thirty days and also doubled the percentage of body fat reduction. Furthermore, one animal study indicated that ashwagandha could reduce cholesterol and triglycerides by as much as 53%. A clinical study with humans indicated a 17% reduction in LDL and an 11% decrease in triglycerides, suggesting supplementation with *Withania somnifera* as a potential alternative to pharmaceutical statin medication.

Synergy between ashwagandha and CBD

The adaptogenic and rejuvenating effects of ashwagandha in tandem with all the many properties of CBD could be a potent combination to aid patients in the reduction of stress and anxiety, for energy boosting, and for treating such issues as depression, insomnia, and chronic pain. Their "homeostasis balancing" double act could be considered a boon to a population seeking a more natural approach.

Both CBD and ashwagandha are considered effective stress reducers, ashwagandha working through the HPA axis (hypothalamus–pituitary–adrenal axis) whereby it acts in maintaining a balance of cortisol and other corticosteroids. It is particularly helpful in cases of exhaustion and stress. Simultaneously CBD would be operating via the endocannabinoid system, centred in the limbic and paralimbic regions of the brain. Combining the two herbs could address all possible causes of stress, each herb synergistically enhancing the performance of the other.

Additionally, the joint action of herbs could be especially useful in the management of chronic pain. While CBD activates the vanilloid receptors to reduce the number of pain signals to the brain and thus increasing pain tolerance, ashwagandha accentuates or enhances CBD's abilities and is found to be particularly helpful in cases of degenerative disc back pain, sciatica, diabetic neuropathy, trigeminal neuralgia, and conditions such as carpal tunnel syndrome.

Other herbs which have shown a proven synergy with cannabis include black pepper, ginger root, white peony root, Chinese angelica (*dong quai*), white willow bark, turmeric, and antioxidant mushrooms such as cordyceps or maitake.

Cannabis and turmeric

Curcuma longa (turmeric) is an incredible antioxidant; it has antibiotic qualities; it is anti-inflammatory; aids digestion; it is anti-obesity and anti-carcinogenic. For some years now turmeric has been touted as the "cure-all" wonder drug on social media, the internet, and in health magazines and articles. It contains curcumin and zingiberene (being in the Zingiber or ginger family). There is now even turmeric tea readily for sale in most supermarkets.

Turmeric stimulates bile flow from the liver and aids digestion, aids detoxification, and can protect the liver against damage (making it a fabulous companion to milk thistle). It can help to regulate the gut flora, so it is good to be taken after antibiotics, and also soothes the gut mucosa. It also has blood sugar lowering properties which makes it particularly useful for diabetics. Additionally, turmeric can lower cholesterol levels and can inhibit blood clotting by the method of blocking prostaglandin production; this means turmeric needs to be taken with great care if on blood thinners. In the respiratory system turmeric enhances immunity and as an antioxidant it protects against damage from free radicals. It is such a good anti-inflammatory that it is immensely helpful for conditions such as arthritis and fibromyalgia, as well as for liver and gall bladder issues.

The combination of turmeric with CBD is a synergistic powerhouse for chronic pain and inflammation. Turmeric also increases the bioavailability of CBD making it more easily assimilated in the body. CBD has inherent anti-anxiety effects and with the added antioxidant and antidepressant qualities of turmeric this makes a winning combination. For conditions such as arthritis, fibromyalgia, polymyalgia, rheumatica and generalised aches and pains the combination of turmeric capsules alongside the CBD has been proven to give fabulous relief to thousands of patients and customers, including myself and members of my own family.

Cannabis and cacao

Theobroma cacao comes from the cocoa bean. The name "theobroma" means "food of the gods" in Latin, and it is antioxidant, helps digestion, increases blood flow to the heart, and elevates the mood—amongst its many other qualities. Cacao contains minute quantities of anandamide, which is the endocannabinoid that is also known as "the happy hormone" and which is naturally produced within the body. It also contains tryptophan, which is a serotonin precursor, which explains why cacao helps to balance the system so well. In Central America, the cocoa bean was used to treat pregnancy problems and for the easing of childbirth. Cacao also contains theobromine, which has similarities to caffeine; additionally, cacao contains xanthines which help relieve and relax bronchial spasms and can therefore be useful for the treatment of allergies and asthma. The use of high quality chocolate with high cacao levels could increase the levels of neurotransmitters such as serotonin and dopamine. It is known that women often crave chocolate around the time of menstruation, which indicates that there may be a hormonal balancing element to chocolate. Cacao does not only contain anandamide, but it also contains, in significant quantities, substances which inhibit the breakdown of cannabinoids such as N-oleolethanolamine (OEA), a weight gain inhibitor, and N-linoleoylethanolamine (NAE), which is an anti-inflammatory molecule. These two metabolites inhibit the breakdown of anandamide and it is posited that they also inhibit the breakdown of cannabinoids such as CBD which means the CBD stays in the system longer.

Combining cacao with CBD not only improves the taste of the CBD—when I offer customers CBD oils or pastes, I often recommend they pop their drop of CBD onto a chocolate button and allow it to melt in the pouch of their cheek—to get absorbed into the mucous membranes. In all honesty, CBD does not taste great, so this is a fabulous way of disguising the taste. But the fats within the chocolate will also enhance bioavailability of the CBD, and the synergistic effects of chocolate or cacao with CBD mean that the mood-elevating, relaxing, pleasurable feelings will thereby be enhanced synergistically.

CHAPTER 11

Cannabis and cancer—The Cancer Act of 1939

The Cancer Act of 1939 prohibits any manufacturer of CBD products (or any herbal product) from making any claims whatsoever with regard to cancer. It states that "No person shall take any part in the publication of any advertisement which … may offer to treat any person for cancer, or to prescribe any remedy therefor, or to give any advice in connection with the treatment thereof." It further clarifies that "In this section the expression 'advertisement' includes any notice, circular, label, wrapper or other document, and any announcement made orally or by any means of producing or transmitting sounds."

Despite this admonition, there is still a huge subculture and inference that CBD or cannabis with THC will "cure" cancer, and this needs to be addressed. There is ongoing research, but thus far clinical trials and publication of findings are scant. Evidently, research continues but finding evidence beyond the anecdotal is harder.

A 2019 review discussed that there was a reasonable amount of evidence and clinical trials to consider cannabis for such conditions as nausea and vomiting, loss of appetite, and pain. Furthermore, there was some promising evidence looking at chemotherapy-induced peripheral neuropathy, gastrointestinal distress, and sleep disorders, but that literature was far too scant to provide clinical evidence. The study concluded that cannabis had "multifaceted potential bioactive benefits" and called for more research to be done.

A further study in 2019 examined the in-vitro effects of CBD on human gastric cancer cells. The study discovered that CBD significantly inhibited the proliferation and colony formation of such cells. The study found that cell apoptosis in gastric cancer was significantly enhanced with the use of CBD and concluded that it might be a valuable tool in the fight against cancer.

A Canadian paper published in 2019 called for action with regard to the fact that many patients are using cannabis to manage symptoms related to cancer and cancer treatment. It raised concerns that patients were accessing cannabis from friends and family or from "casual or unlicensed suppliers". The paper discussed the fact that the public are "inundated with media stories" about cannabis and its potential as a cure-all. The author called for more work regarding "furthering the science of cannabis as it pertains to cancer care".

With regard to personal and anecdotal experiences using CBD with cancer patients, I have seen some amazing results. This is not to say that it works for every person, it does not, and it is not the miracle that completely removes cancer—while helping the person feel "better in themselves", have a little more energy, feel less nausea, get a better night's sleep, and in some cases ease their breathing, or increase their appetite.

I have had several amazing recoveries, where patients using CBD alongside chemotherapy have made recoveries—although it is entirely possible that because they had chemotherapy so "of course" that is what must have cured them—but often people undergoing these treatments suffer noteworthy side effects—the patients I have seen that used CBD concomitantly with chemotherapy all had significantly fewer negative side effects.

CHAPTER 12

Studies on the effects of CBD in pets

As discussed at the beginning of this book, animals, like humans, have an endocannabinoid system. So, therefore, it follows that what works for the human endocannabinoid system could equally well work for pets.

A study published in *Frontiers in Veterinary Science* in July 2018 looks at the pharmacokinetics, safety, and efficacy of CBD treatment in dogs suffering from arthritis. A clinical trial was performed in which a selection of dogs suffering from osteoarthritis were given CBD. Half of the group were given a placebo. It was observed that the dogs given the CBD appeared to experience significantly less pain than the placebo group. The dogs in the CBD group were more active and experienced no side effects. There were issues with various delivery vehicles of the medication. Those dogs given the product in a powdered capsule did not react as well as the dogs given the product within an oil base. It was felt that owing to the lipophilic nature of CBD, an oil-based vehicle provided preferable and more consistent results. The lipophilic nature of CBD means it is enhanced when delivered alongside a fat, or fat-containing food. The study further discussed the conditions the pet owners felt could be relieved by the ingestion of CBD, including pain, inflammation, anxiety and phobia, digestive system issues, and pruritis. Other studies they evaluated after their trial discussed the effects of CBD upon immune-mediated and inflammatory allergic disorders in dogs as well as its anti-convulsant and anti-epileptic effects in dogs. The study concludes that owing to the fact that different strains of cannabis produce differing amounts of CBD and other related cannabinoids, their findings may not translate to products other than the one used in the study, due to the differing cannabinoid concentrations in a "largely unregulated market".

A 2012 study using rats and mice suffering from chronic inflammation resulted in evidence that the animals given the CBD had significantly lower levels of inflammation after a course of treatment.

A neurologist at Colorado State University, Dr Stephanie McGrath, performed a clinical trial which evidenced that 89% of dogs treated with CBD experienced fewer epileptic seizures. She stated that "Overall, what we found seems very promising."

The explosion of the CBD industry in the UK and certain states in America, also Canada and some European countries, means that people successfully using CBD to alleviate some of their conditions are interested in whether this can help their pets. The UK, in particular, is a nation of animal lovers! Many people treat their pets better than they treat themselves and there has been a surge in healthier foods, grain-free and raw diets, and treats which now include botanicals for the health of the nation's pets. As any creature with a backbone has an endocannabinoid system, this means that reptiles, amphibians, fish, birds, and mammals, including our common house pets, cats, dogs, and rabbits, could respond well to CBD.

The great majority of the evidence is anecdotal, although while running a health shop and working in a CBD store I found that many customers used CBD for their pets. There have been significant success stories too, and a few sad cases. One such case was that of a dog, whose owner came into our shop in tears. Their dog, merely four years old, had been having seizures for some time. On the day before they walked into our shop, the dog had had over fifteen seizures and the vet had to be called. The vet had told the owners that he felt the dog may be best put to sleep as it was unfair on the dog and the owners to go through this trauma. The seizures were becoming more regular and stronger each time. The dog was by this point having seizures almost daily, although admittedly not usually more than fifteen in a day. It was our first case of the owners of a dog coming in and asking for something for their pet. We explained to the owners that strictly speaking we do not "prescribe" for pets, but the owners were insistent they wanted to try something, anything to prolong the life of their beloved pet. We agreed to let the owner take a small tube of CBD paste and suggested a small rice grain-sized amount be administered to the dog. This was on a Monday. On the Friday they telephoned the shop to say that the dog had been completely seizure free from Monday through to Friday; however, on Friday afternoon the dog had a tiny seizure. I recommended increasing the dosage and giving two rice grain size pieces a day. From that day for the next three months the dog had no seizures. The customers became regulars, each time more ebullient and joyful that their dog was so much better and "behaving like a puppy again". After three months the dog had a further seizure and once more the dosage was increased slightly. The dog survived a further three months, but sadly had a significant seizure and had to be put to sleep. The owners came into the shop and we wept together. One feels so terribly helpless and somehow to "blame". As a healer, one does just want to heal everyone. However, the owner expressed her gratitude. She told me, "Without the cannabis paste, our dog would have been dead months ago. We had many more months with her than we expected, and her quality of life was so improved."

Since that day, many more customers have come to the shop, seeking CBD for their pets. From dogs, cats, to even rabbits, and for conditions such as arthritis and pain, inflammation, anxiety and stress, to calm them down; epilepsy and seizures, gastrointestinal disorders, neurodegenerative conditions, sleep disorders, and also for dogs with cancerous growths or skin conditions. In almost every case, there has been an improvement in the animal's condition, irrespective of what it is.

With regard to dogs, it is interesting to note that dogs actually have more cannabinoid receptors in their brains than humans, suggesting that dogs could be particularly responsive to cannabis and CBD.

As dogs salivate more heavily than humans, it is better to ingest CBD than to try to rub it onto their gums (if the dog were to let you). Provided that it is mixed with a fat it will be more effective and bioavailable. As with humans the dosage should be extremely low to start with and very slowly and gradually increased until the dog appears to be pain free or symptom free. CBD does appear to be very well tolerated by dogs based on anecdotal examples and as it is completely non-toxic it should not do any harm.

Actually, that is an interesting point to mention. At no time has anyone ever suffered a fatal dose of cannabis—the same cannot be said for pharmaceuticals. Even paracetamol can cause liver damage and with over ingestion risk fatal outcomes. The amount of CBD the body would need to ingest to cause a fatal dose has not yet been discovered in any research that I can find.

As a health food shop owner and medical herbalist I am not qualified to prescribe for pets, and what an owner does with the products we sell is really up to them. We did make it clear to every customer that we were not qualified in veterinary practice. However, when faced with desperate owners that wanted suggestions for what they could use, we were able to give advice as to what would alleviate pain with humans.

CHAPTER 13

What to look for when purchasing CBD?

I can really only discuss the UK marketplace here, as that is what I know; I have not purchased or sought CBD in other countries. Companies I have worked with have organic products and know the source of their raw product. My current employer sources the hand cleaned, outdoor grown raw material from a certified organic farm in the Czech Republic, imports the products into the UK, and then uses super critical carbon-dioxide extraction method to produce high-grade broad-spectrum oils. Each product comes with its own certificate of analysis for each batch that is made—this is extremely important. If the company you are buying from does not have a genuine certificate of analysis for each product then you should avoid them.

Colour is not necessarily an indicator of quality—so if the product is thick, tarry, and black, or light and golden, that does not necessarily mean it is not good quality (although previously this may have been the case). The reason some products are lighter than others depends upon the extraction methods, and whether chlorophyll and other plant materials are extracted. The cheapest products on the market are often made from "isolates", that is to say an isolated CBD without any other phytochemicals. These are manufactured in large quantities in Eastern Europe and America and are often extremely cheap to buy in; they then just require bottling and labelling so each company looks "individual". These inferior products are flooding the UK marketplace. The problem is they come with few instructions, no contraindications, and often highly inaccurate or completely lacking information. People use these products, find that they get no results, and dismiss the product as ineffective or useless.

I have run a health shop since 2014 and gradually my suppliers started selling CBD products. Initially, there was an American imported flavoured CBD oil, which was quickly followed by a UK produced CBD spray, and then the market became deluged. It seemed everyone and their dog was selling, producing, or marketing some form of CBD oil. It had become the "panacea" to cure all ills. Whilst I passionately believe that this is a wonderful addition to an herbalist's arsenal, it cannot work on all the levels that a multi-herb approach can. Nevertheless, it is important to know what to look for when buying these products.

As discussed in the previous paragraph a lot of products on the market are "ready to go", purchased in from Eastern Europe or the United States. There is no guarantee of organic; there is no indication of which chemicals were used to extract the oil—that is a minefield in itself—and there is no parity across descriptions. Some describe their product in milligrams, some in percentages, some in both.

The strengths vary across the brands. Some label themselves as "extra high strength" but when you examine the packaging closely you will see that this can be as little as 2% CBD oil, so please ensure you read all labelling carefully before committing to purchasing something. The prices can also vary wildly. Some products of extremely low quality are being sold for more than £70 for a 10 ml bottle of oil. Using sources like eBay is not recommended as you have no idea who is selling a product you are planning to ingest. A laboratory report done by a company I worked for found that an oil selling on eBay as a CBD oil was in fact hemp seed cooking oil, bottled into little 10 ml dropper bottles and selling for in excess of £35 a bottle.

Check the company website. Do they offer laboratory reports on their product guaranteeing the CBD content of each batch? Do they list where they source their raw material from? Do they offer a "sample" system, whereby you can buy for a discount a sample bottle of their oil to see what you think of the quality and efficacy?

Before deciding upon which product to buy, think about various things. Important to consider is the delivery method—there are so many different delivery methods of CBD available and what suits one person may not suit another. Please refer to the next chapter regarding delivery methods.

Consider the effect you might be looking for. Do you need something energising and for the day-time? Or would you rather it was relaxing and soporific and would help to sleep for the night-time? Is it for pain relief or for inflammation? CBD by its very nature is anti-inflammatory so reduction in inflammation is pretty much guaranteed whichever product you choose.

Consider the colour, the smell, and taste of the product. Most good quality CBD can smell rather pungent and taste quite strong—someone described it to me as tasting the way BabyBio (a plant fertiliser) smells!

Some CBD oils are flavoured to disguise the taste of the oil—that is not necessarily a bad thing depending upon what type of flavouring has been used. If it is a natural flavouring from plant terpenes or plant extracts, that is not such a bad thing. If the product is evidently a synthetically flavoured product, I, personally, would avoid it.

When starting to take a product, "low and slow" is the way to go! Take an extremely small dose, regularly for about a week—this may be as low as one or two drops a day. After a week, you may increase the dosage by one drop, again for one week. In the third week you can increase the dosage by one drop again—until you start seeing an effect. There is a pictorial description of how to dose in the next chapter. It can take a considerable time for the endocannabinoid system to kick in and for effects to be noticed, several months in some cases, so be persistent. This is not a "pharmaceutical" product which blocks pain receptors and acts in twenty minutes. This is a natural food supplement that enhances the body's own inflammatory responses and can alleviate certain conditions very effectively, provided the consumer is patient. If you are a practitioner giving the product to a patient—you (and they) may think that the condition is extremely severe and therefore needs the strongest product. I have lost count of the times a patient has asked me for "the strongest thing you've got please". It is important you do not make the mistake of falling into this trap—an excess of CBD will fool the body's receptors into thinking there is too much, and receptors will close off. Too much, too quickly floods the system and there will be little or no efficacious effect.

It is a good idea to keep a log or note of how much you have taken and when. During my time working in health stores, we would often get customers after a week or ten days telling us "it's not working" and we would ask them to persist. After a few months, they often, of their own accord, think they are better and they do not need their CBD product any more, or they think it is not doing much. Studies show that the improvement in health is very gradual and almost unnoticeable. Just as one becomes accustomed to having a certain level of pain, conversely, a person becomes accustomed to having less pain—as this is a gradual process after a few months they think it is not doing much. So, they stop taking it. A week to ten days later they will be back in the shop asking for their product. They notice after a little while that their symptoms begin to return—and it is at this point they realise how much the CBD was helping with their aches and pains.

Every person is unique, their endocannabinoid system is unique and reacts uniquely to the product, and their condition is unique to them. I often tell people, "You are your body's best doctor." One knows oneself better than anyone else who is not inside one's body. Therefore, it really is up to each individual patient to tailor a dose to something that suits them.

There is no risk of overdose. If you swallowed an entire bottle of CBD, it is unlikely that anything negative is going to happen to you beyond perhaps feeling very tired and needing to rest. However, in all cases, I recommend ensuring that you seek the advice of a qualified medical herbalist or other professional who has trained in herbs and their application before commencing a programme of CBD ingestion.

CHAPTER 14

Delivery methods and contraindications

There are four basic delivery methods of taking CBD—inhalation, oral ingestion, sublingual, and topical either with a salve, or more recently skin patches. Anal suppositories are also sometimes available and in certain cases these can be a real benefit to a patient who is unable for one reason or another to ingest the product.

Inhalation

There are now shops in London selling "wraps", a CBD rich THC low "cigarette" that people can smoke. This would not be my personal preference for delivery owing to the side effects of smoke inhalation and whether tobacco is or isn't included and the potential carcinogenic effects of this.

Vaporising—vaping—is becoming enormously popular and there are a series of very high-quality CBD vape products available on the market. Some of these contain additional terpenes for added medicinal benefit. I know of at least one product that is created not using the PG/VG (propylene glycol/vegetable glycerine) method of dispersal but using pure terpenes as the delivery agent. The advantage of vaping is that the onset of pain relief or other relief is very swift, within minutes. Because it has such a rapid effect, it is easier to dose to ensure that the maximum benefit is achieved, and it is (arguably) healthier than smoking. The effects of vaping CBD last between one and four hours but can then be repeated. So, one would not be vaping CBD in the same way one would vape another oil—one would use one or two drags every four hours or so.

Nebulisers—obviously smoking and vaping carry with them a variety of health risks, and thus very recently, nebulisers have begun to appear on the market as a safe, clean alternative to vaping. A nebuliser works by pushing compressed air through a compartment filled with CBD oil. As the air moves at an extremely high velocity through the oil, it turns into an aerosol spray which may be inhaled by the patient. Many asthmatics will recognise the nebuliser which is usually used to administer salbutamol, which relaxes the muscles of the airways which makes it easier to breathe. There is no residue or lingering odour with nebulised CBD and little to no taste (although I have seen fruit flavoured CBD products aimed at nebulisers). There have been very few studies on nebulisers alongside CBD and bioavailability in order to confirm specific absorption percentages—partly because hitherto it has not been possible to nebulise CBD. As CBD is hydrophobic, it does not "dissolve" in water; however, for many years scientists have been working on how to make hydrophobic compounds water soluble. This has become far more viable in recent years with advances in technology and there are now several ways that it is possible to create a water-soluble CBD. A nano emulsion involves adding microscopic droplets of CBD into a substance it is typically incapable of dissolving in; this keeps it from separating from water when mixed together. Microemulsions are similar to nano emulsions but with slightly larger droplets. Creating a liposomal CBD is another possibility but is a difficult process requiring high levels of surfactants and expensive equipment in order to process this. There are also micellar products, water dispersible liquids containing cannabinoids or water-soluble powder consisting of maltodextrin powder coated with broad spectrum oil, dispersible in water.

However, although the mechanism of inhaling through a nebuliser is similar to using a vaporiser, a large difference is that the water compounds from a mist will deliver almost 100% of the CBD to the lungs whereas vaping will result in a loss of CBD and prove much costlier in the long run. It is therefore sensible to extrapolate that bioavailability is far higher in a nebuliser than in a vaporiser.

Oral ingestion

There are a wide variety of CBD edibles on the market now, from gummies to chocolate to brownies and more. However, to me, using food to deliver the product does not allow for a specifically tailored dose. It is also possible to have CBD capsules, and many companies are now providing these in various strengths. It is always best to start on the lowest dose and work your way up the dosage range, rather than start on the strongest, for reasons previously mentioned. Flooding the endocannabinoid system with too much cannabinoid will simply induce the CBD to "switch" the receptors off, and there will be no real benefit.

Capsules take effect after about one to two hours, peaking at around three to four hours, and appear to last for around six to eight hours in the body. It is more difficult to dose, as one does not feel an effect immediately, so it is difficult for the patient to gauge how much is required. The advantage of a capsule is that it is generally a set standard dose in each capsule, so the consumer always knows how much they are getting. With oils it is difficult to gauge unless you are extremely precise, which many people are not. However, there is no nasty taste, which is a complaint of the oils and in some cases with the vapes. There is no "equipment" required; the capsule is a complete package on its own. It is a very discreet way to take the product; no one around can tell what you are taking.

Sublingual

Using a dropper bottle or a spray bottle—both are readily available on the marketplace today—a certain number of drops (or sprays) are squirted under the tongue. With the dropper bottle this can be tricky for some, especially the elderly, as the dosage must be accurate and low. The tendency for people to not bother to count the number of drops and simply squirt an entire dropper full under their tongue is high. It is often best to perform this action in front of a mirror—the important part is the product needs to be kept in contact with the oral mucosa for around two minutes if possible—so therefore, needs to be held under the tongue for around two minutes before swallowing. This is to allow the product to be absorbed by the mucous membranes in the mouth and thus be transferred into the bloodstream avoiding the gut and first pass of the liver.

If there is difficulty getting the drops into the mouth, then I have often suggested using a chocolate button or piece of chocolate to count drops onto, then popping it into the pouch of the cheek and letting it dissolve.

The onset of effect is usually in around fifteen minutes to half an hour and can last from about an hour up to six hours. It is now possible to get sublingual strips, although this presentation may only be available for the US marketplace.

Topical application

Many companies are now manufacturing creams, salves, oils, gels, and lotions for topical application. These are for external skin use only. They can be applied as needed to areas of pain, or to skin conditions—both have been helped by CBD rich products. CBD absorbs particularly well through the skin and both on its own and with the addition of other plant extracts, essential oils, or butters, it can be extremely helpful for a wide range of conditions. It is wise to always test on a small inconspicuous area of skin before using a topical application just to ensure there is no allergic reaction. The topical application can have a multitude of uses. In my own practice I tend to make my own creams and add CBD oil into a cream and mix it thoroughly, with some astounding results. My daughter suffers from extreme migraines, owing to head trauma, and these can continue for hours and hours with intermittent vomiting and extreme pain. Using a calendula-based cream with some added CBD and some essential oil of lavender, this migraine can lift in less than an hour. We have tried this method repeatedly and it has worked every time. She feels it's "magical".

Skin patches are a new consideration and I believe the company for whom I currently work may be the only ones selling these skin patches in the UK, although these are far more common in the United States. By putting on a skin patch with concentrated CBD that releases through the skin in time, this negates the need for ingestion or sublingual application and may become a very common choice in time, especially with the popularity of the nicotine patches which have helped so many people give up smoking. The skin patch will give targeted and specific cannabis dosage. There should be few or no side effects, which allows for a more concentrated dosage—an unobtrusive yet effective distribution method.

Research indicates that skin patches interact with the transcutaneous endocannabinoid system and may enter the bloodstream—however, because they are not digested, they by-pass the digestive tract and liver, avoiding the "first pass" CYP450 interactions, therefore there should be no interaction with existing prescription medications when using a topical product. However, there could potentially be an allergic reaction (not to the CBD but to the adhesive used in the patch) so it is considered prudent to cut a small part of a patch and place it on the inside of the wrist for twenty-four hours to ensure there is no allergic reaction.

For ease of reference I have included an image overleaf which gives a graphical representation of how to take the oils.

How to take CBD oil

It is wise to start slowly with cannabis oil, personalising the dosage by gradually increasing the number of drops taken until the desired results are attained. This approach allows you to tailor the amount of cannabis oil your patient/client takes to fit in with their personal needs without confusing or overloading their endocannabinoid system.

We are all individuals and as such may require different approaches, so it is important you encourage your clients to allow their body to be its own best doctor—this is only a guideline and some people may require a slower approach, increasing the dose each fortnight. This guide is merely an example of

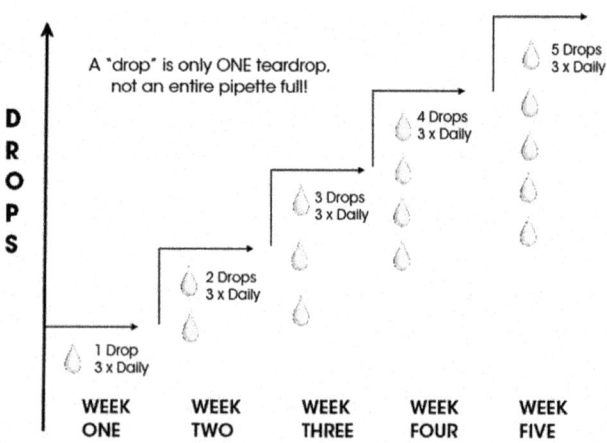

If they are taking a daytime and night-time product, then use the daytime product for the first two doses and the night-time product for the last, night-time dose.

how you could approach dosage. To reiterate, it is always best to start low and slow to allow the endocannabinoid system to "wake up" and give your client the benefit they are looking for. Once you find the right dose for their needs, there is no need to continue increasing, simply continue with that dosage.

It may take a few weeks for the endocannabinoid system to react, but overdoing the cannabis oil is also unhelpful as it confuses the cannabinoid receptors in the body. Start with a low dose every time, do not be tempted because you feel their condition is particularly bad to start with a higher dose, this simply floods the system and will not work.

CBD interactions with other herbs or pharmaceuticals

It is vitally important to take special note of CBD–herb–drug interactions—CBD interacts with *every* other drug, because it operates through the enzymatic pathway CYP450, and the associated family of enzymes, because it has a tendency to take up the entire bandwidth of the pathway or attach itself to other herbs or drugs to enhance or even block their actions. CBD must always be taken separately from all other pharmaceuticals and some herbals. That is, there should be at least a two-hour gap between minor pharmaceuticals and a four-hour gap between CBD and a major drug such as morphine—and that includes co-codamol or codeine. Strangely enough, grapefruit also affects the same enzymatic pathway, so if a medicine states that one cannot ingest grapefruit or grapefruit products while taking this medicine, then it stands to reason that one should also not be taking CBD.

The issue of morphine patches is an extremely tricky one, because it is a topical application it should not interact through CYP-450, however, the interaction between CBD and morphine is strong, and therefore, I would not recommend using CBD concomitantly with morphine patches unless closely monitored by a health professional who is trained in CBD.

The issue is that when more than one "drug" or supplement uses the cytochrome P450 pathway they interact with each other. The metabolism of all drugs can be affected, inhibited, or potentiated when taken concomitantly. The more "drugs" or medicines a person takes, the more complicated the interactions will be. CBD is a potent inhibitor of other drugs and when taken with competing medicines CBD will elbow other drugs out of the way to be used first, which can reduce the effectiveness of other medications.

Drugs which also use the CYP450 enzyme system are as follows:

- Steroids
- HMG-CoA reductase inhibitors
- Calcium channel blockers
- Antihistamines
- Prokinetics
- HIV antivirals
- Immune modulators
- Anti-arrhythmic drugs
- Anaesthetics
- Anti-epileptics
- Beta-blockers
- Proton pump inhibitors (PPIs)
- Non-steroidal anti-inflammatory drugs (NSAIDs)
- Angiotensin II blockers
- Oral hypoglycaemic agents
- Sulfonylureas
- Contraceptive Pill.

Antibiotics

It is a good idea to let the doctor know if taking antibiotics on the same day as taking CBD. There has been no research to show that there is any interaction with antibiotics, but using the gap between taking them should at least prevent any negative side effects.

Chemotherapy

Interestingly, CBD appears to interact with chemotherapy but in a positive way. There is also some data suggesting that CBD in high doses interacts positively with radiation therapy. It can certainly help ameliorate the effects of chemotherapy, by reducing nausea and pain and feelings of low mood and depression as well as slightly increasing the appetite. Many patients on chemotherapy have reported that upon adding CBD into their daily routine their appetite has returned.

Antidepressants and anti-anxiety medicines

There is no clear research to state whether CBD interacts negatively with antidepressants, antipsychotics, or benzodiazepines; however, they do use the CYP450 pathway, and also interact with serotonin and dopamine in the brain, so a sensible four-hour gap between taking this type of medication and CBD is recommended. It is important to tell the main health care practitioner if using CBD as well as medicines in this group.

Blood thinners

Some blood thinners are a problem in that they do interact with CBD, specifically warfarin and clopidogrel. If taking those medications, it is wise to avoid CBD completely, and they should not be considered at all without a full consultation with a doctor or primary health care practitioner. However, heparin and factor xa inhibitors are considered safe to combine with CBD, although again the four-hour gap between administration is recommended.

Ibuprofen

Once more, unfortunately, there is little research into interactions between CBD and ibuprofen; however, it does use the same enzymatic pathway for its metabolisation, so leaving at least a two-hour gap is recommended. This could also be dependent upon how sensitive the patient/person taking the CBD and ibuprofen is—I, for example, have taken CBD and ibuprofen too close together: the first time I did this by accident and I felt quite "jolly" and a little uninhibited—similar to the feeling one has after drinking a glass of alcohol but not to the point of being drunk. However, as a practitioner it is wise to advise patients to leave that gap just in case they have a reaction to it.

Topical CBD

If using a prescription topical cream or ointment and then using a CBD product topically there should be no real issue. Topical products are not subject to P450 degradation, so they will not interact with the same pathway in the liver. However, a patch test is always recommended when using any topical product for the first time.

CHAPTER 15

Health conditions and their responses to CBD

The most important thing to bear in mind with CBD is that it balances—it aims to create homeostasis within the body. Everybody seeks balance, whether that be a mind and body balance, a work–life balance, or a balance in their relationships, immune systems, or even in their diet!

The body itself seeks balance, or homeostasis—a stable internal environment and this depends upon a huge variety of variables within the body's own systems, whether that be blood pressure, temperature, or blood glucose levels, thyroid levels, sex hormone levels, mental health levels—the list goes on—the body wants to be balanced!

The endocannabinoid system, as previously discussed, manages all the diverse body systems and can therefore impact upon every aspect of health. With regard to dosing, this is a tricky question because the endocannabinoid system is genetically different in each individual. The amount of CBD required varies from person to person and this is also dependent upon the endocannabinoid system being "balanced". If it is slightly imbalanced the effects of CBD can vary dramatically from one patient to the next.

Priming the endocannabinoid system

The one thing we always tell customers and patients is to start on the very lowest dose, "low and slow", to encourage the endocannabinoid system gently to do its work. There is absolutely no point in starting on a high dose because the consumer feels their condition is "so bad" that it must require the strongest possible product to alleviate it. Starting on such a high dose will simply encourage the cannabinoid receptors to close off, and will not give the consumer or user a good result.

Conditions

I have seen CBD help an incredibly wide variety of conditions, and often people who come to see me are "at the end of the road"—they have tried everything else and they come to see me because nothing else has worked. Then they expect a miraculous cure within a week, because they have read an article telling them that CBD is the new "wonder" supplement.

The range of scientific studies into various conditions is extremely limited. There are so many variables when studying cannabis and the endocannabinoid system that it makes it extremely difficult to get consistency and good "p" values when doing scientific research. Although animals also have an endocannabinoid system, the way that it works in an animal may differ from how it works in a human and so it is difficult to compare these results to human physiology. However, most of the research I have found has been using mouse or rat models. Different plant chemovars can also vary, because it is not just the CBD content that is important: the other phytochemicals present in that particular plant also play an important role. This can change depending upon the growing conditions of the plant, what it was fed during growth, what was the constitution of the soil the plant was grown in, its provenance, whether it was exposed to sunlight or LED lights, and many other factors.

All these variables affect the consistency of any study. Any group of humans participating in a study will all have various levels of endocannabinoid deficiency or dysfunction, which also makes it hard to calculate accurate outcomes.

What I have seen in practice is remarkable: each patient has a different experience, but predominantly these have been extremely good. The preponderance of chronic ailments have very similar symptoms; these are chronic pain, inflammation, sleep disruption, anxiety and low mood; loss of "joy" is one I often hear. People would come in to see me asking for "the one for arthritis please" or "the one for fibromyalgia". I explain patiently to each person that CBD does not work like this. It is generally anti-inflammatory—so all inflammatory conditions should see some benefits. Different chemovars can be mood-elevating or energising, whilst others can be soporific and relaxing. The net result is that CBD can help manage these symptoms and whilst it's not a cure for any particular condition, it alleviates the symptoms so very successfully that the person is no longer as hampered by their condition as they were before. But it is worth noting that these symptoms will return if the person stops taking the cannabis. However, on the upside, cannabis is far less harmful to a person than the vast majority of pharmaceutical preparations, so that must be a good thing. Almost every patient I have seen, and I have treated or dealt with in excess of 6000 patients and customers in the past few years, has experienced some benefit. They are no longer suffering and are able to continue with their lives in a way they could not before they took their CBD supplement. It is true, it has not worked for every single person—but they really are only a handful—and often those people who are of the "more is better" school of thought, and who have simply taken far too much CBD and thereby flooded their system. There are also that element who think that "nothing will work", and it is interesting to note that sometimes in those people, it does indeed not work— I find that fascinating and have often wondered about the "positive mental attitude" towards health and life in general—feeling that people who have such negative emotions hamper their own recovery, which must be down to brain chemicals.

Pain relief

This is possibly one of the most important things, to me, that CBD can do. The number of people I have seen daily who reported that they had a new lease of life! Customers and patients who used to come to see me on crutches and who are after about a month on CBD came to see me without those crutches; people who could no longer walk very far, coming to tell me they were now able to take the dog on long beach walks and their knees didn't hurt any more. It has been such a joy to talk to people daily who thank you for helping them get rid of their pain. Many people I have seen were able to reduce or stop taking the high strength prescription medicines they were taking after they started their journey. People have found that when the pain has been relieved there is an impact on every area of their life. Their mood becomes improved, life becomes generally easier, anxiety is reduced, and sleep also generally improves. There is some useful research on the reduction of neuropathic pain, pain after chemotherapy, chronic pain, and so forth. Some studies have used animal models, which as previously mentioned may not be a completely accurate way of establishing how a human being reacts to a cannabinoid. However, I can speak from personal experience of the thousands of now pain-free individuals I have treated, who are no longer taking tramadol, or ibuprofen, or other opioid painkillers and who are enjoying their life significantly more than before they commenced their CBD journey.

A woman patient, sixty-nine years old, but remarkably young for her age, came to see me. She had been suffering from high blood pressure and as she finally admitted to me an addiction to high strength pain killers (tramadol). At one point, she admitted she had been taking at least eight or more a day. She had through self-care and yoga managed to halve this number but could not get off her dose of four tramadol daily. There were other underlying issues; she suffered from insomnia and had been on antidepressants in the past but did not want to go back onto these. The patient also suffered from several other conditions including tinnitus, insomnia, and postnasal drip. In addition to the herbal prescription I devised for her, I suggested she try CBD to see if we could improve her pain levels.

After one month on CBD, she was able to reduce her tramadol use down gradually and by the fifth week was not using tramadol at all. Despite not resolving the postnasal drip, the tinnitus was markedly improved. The patient finally reverted to only a CBD regimen, and following her consultation often came to see me to tell me how much improved she felt. She was completely free of her "addiction" to painkillers, which had been ongoing for around fifteen years and was absolutely delighted.

Attention deficit disorder and attention deficit hyperactivity disorder

I have lots of patients and customers both adults and children who suffer from ADD or ADHD. Often such patients are prescribed pharmaceuticals which will target the dopamine and serotonin balance in the brain, or the norepinephrine also known as noradrenaline which functions as a hormone and neurotransmitter both in the brain and body. I have seen CBD prove especially useful for these patients, in calming down their thought processes and allowing them to manage their day to day tasks. With children, I have used a water soluble based product in a juice, which also has made a significant impact on those children's lives.

As a foster carer of some twenty years, I have fostered a lot of children with ADHD, attachment disorder, and autistic tendencies. The local authority would never have allowed me to use CBD with a child; however, had I had that option I strongly feel that a lot of these children's lives would have been improved dramatically. During my years of practice I have often seen many parents who have been at their wit's end because their child is suffering. Often, such children are not able to go to school because their behaviour is so difficult owing to ADHD or similar conditions. It was especially gratifying to see those parents come back to see me with their success stories. In one particular case, the patient was a child who had not been to school in over six months, yet after three months on CBD found that they were able to concentrate, they were no longer having irascible "outbursts" or rage and anger episodes, and the parents and child both felt this product had completely changed their lives.

Anxiety, stress, and depression

It is truly remarkable how many of us suffer from anxiety. Apart from pain, I think it is the most prevalent issue that people have come to see me with—many times I would hear the same stories—I have anxiety, what can I take that will stop it? People have told me they were suffering from palpitations, a feeling of dread, chest pains, shortness of breath, a sick nauseous feeling in the pit of their stomach, panic attacks, and dizziness. This array of symptoms can have a most serious impact on a person's life. Previously outgoing jolly people become introverted, shy, and reclusive.

Stress is another thing in modern times that almost everyone suffers from. Almost everyone you speak to tells you that they are "stressed". Sometimes stress is a good thing; it is a response to factors in daily life, pressures, deadlines, etc., and what happens is that the adrenal glands release adrenaline which activates the body's defence mechanisms. This causes rapid heart rate, raised blood pressure, pupil dilation, and muscular contraction—ready to spring away from that tiger— it is known as the fight or flight response. Sometimes stress can make you react positively, to jump away from a dangerous situation, or pull your hand away from the flame that is about to burn it. But when stress is a constant factor, this can become anxiety and turn into a feeling of dread, apprehension, and fear. This may be without apparent cause and many patients tell me they have no idea why they feel so anxious, but nevertheless they do. If this level of stress and then anxiety does not resolve itself for whatever reason, this can turn into chronic anxiety, which is a far darker and more dangerous animal. Chronic anxiety can lead to significant mental health issues, deep depression, inability to function normally or even talk or socialise with others. Simple daily tasks and decisions become insurmountable. Some people may be more susceptible to stress than others, some falling apart and declining whilst others thrive on pressure situations.

Excessive anxiety can cause any or all of the following conditions: diarrhoea, dry mouth, rapid heartbeat or palpitations— that feeling that your heart is in your throat, insomnia, irritability or anger, inability to concentrate, feelings of "going mad", and what I call "feeling outside yourself"—not in control of your own actions.

It is also possible that pharmaceutical or recreational drugs could lead to such symptoms owing to side effects or withdrawal—these include alcohol, nicotine, caffeine, some of the ingredients in cough and cold remedies, bronchodilators for asthma, antidepressants, antipsychotics, ADHD medicines, thyroid medicines, diet pills, and the recreational drugs such as cocaine or amphetamines. Having had a recent experience with steroids, I feel I need to add steroids to this list—after some significant pressure from my GP I was asked to take a long-term dose of steroids; however, I reacted so badly to these that after a few months I asked if I could stop taking them. I was told that this had to be done very gradually, by 1mg every four to six weeks. I think coming off steroids is possibly the hardest thing I have ever had to do: the feelings of brain fog, complete exhaustion, and stress as well as irritability that these caused felt insurmountable. Fortunately, with the help of a regular CBD regimen, which I believe helped me through this dark period, I was able to stop taking this invidious medicine.

Anxiety, stress, and depression can have a lifelong impact and seem almost insuperable, but I have seen more and more patients dealing far more effectively with their symptoms with the use of CBD.

I had a patient who was actually considering giving up her job because she was so anxious about going to work, and despite having completely changed her diet, and having followed a rigorous exercise regime to increase her energy levels and endorphins, she was getting to the point where she thought enough was enough. She was a timid patient, and felt she was disregarded at work. We commenced with an herbal regime to support her through the entire process and then added in some CBD capsules for both the morning and the evening. Within six weeks, this particular patient was telling me that her anxiety was almost gone, she was no longer considering giving up her job, and that she was sleeping better, her palpitations were gone, and she appeared more confident and outgoing. After a few months the woman came to see me to tell me that she had felt confident enough to apply for a more senior role in a different company, had been accepted, and was looking forward to a new work life; on a personal note she had joined a gym, she had made some new friends, and was enjoying evenings out at "crowded nightclubs"—previously completely unthinkable.

A thirty-eight-year-old female patient came to see me, suffering from extreme stress and anxiety; her relationship was failing owing to her low mood and outbursts, she suffered from lack of energy, and was always cold. She had previously been a sufferer of anorexia nervosa although this was now resolved. It was clear there were still emotional issues with this patient. Initially, I treated her as an herbal patient, with an herbal prescription in combination with CBD oil. She found the oil extremely unpalatable, and so we exchanged this for capsules. Within four weeks she felt she no longer wished to take the herbal tincture, but wanted to continue with CBD capsules, however. After four months she was in complete remission of all symptoms. Her anxiety was under control; she felt happier and more level-headed. She was now experiencing a full night's sleep and no longer tossing and turning or waking up midway through the night and over-thinking things. She looked so much healthier, almost "glowing". Her IBS had also significantly improved.

Historically, cannabis has been used for thousands of years to help alleviate anxiety and depressive states. It is important to note that a product high in THC could exacerbate these conditions as there is evidence to show that whilst it is relaxing, an excess of THC can cause paranoia, anxiety, and depression with continued use in some people. However, using a CBD rich product, with a variety of terpenes to give balance, is an incredible tool in the arsenal against anxiety and depression.

Arthritis

There are many different types of arthritis, osteoarthritis, rheumatoid arthritis, psoriatic arthritis, and even viral arthritis. The one thing they all have in common is joint pain and stiffness. Pain on waking and "getting going" in the mornings, pain on rising from a seat, pain on walking upstairs, pain on walking anywhere. In time there can be a significant degeneration in the joints, and this causes further problems.

Rheumatoid arthritis

This autoimmune condition happens when the immune system attacks the body's own cells, causing inflammation, stiff and painful joints, and this usually affects the hands, feet, and wrists. It appears to be a cyclical condition, having periods of remission and periods when it "flares up". There is not only a genetic predisposition to rheumatoid arthritis but there is also a dietary element to this condition: poor digestion and constipation can contribute to an accumulation of toxins in the gut and once circulated around the body, this can cause dis-ease—inflammation and degeneration of cartilage.

I have probably seen more people with arthritis and related conditions than any other condition (anxiety has come a close second). Many of the patients who came to see me for a consultation were on a veritable plethora of different drugs and medications to try to resolve their issues. The vast majority of them have found significant improvement with the ingestion of CBD although I tend to always offer a turmeric supplement in addition to the CBD. As discussed in Chapter 9, the synergistic action of the turmeric and CBD works incredibly well to reduce inflammation and by reducing inflammation the pain is significantly improved. Both CBD and turmeric have pain relieving (nociceptive) qualities, which of course adds to their effectiveness.

Some research has shown that cannabinoid therapy can provide symptomatic relief of joint pain and swelling as well as halting the progression of the disease and the destruction of the joints in question.

In my experience with patients and customers, what has worked most effectively is a combination of different type products; for example, a daytime energising CBD and a night-time relaxing, more soporific CBD, both of which have anti-inflammatory properties, not only allow the person to start enjoying their life, able to do things they could not do before, but also then get a decent night's sleep.

One particularly heart-warming tale of the benefits of CBD oil was of an elderly woman who hadn't been able to knit for more than five years owing to the arthritis in her fingers.

She had tried pharmaceutical medications, pain relievers, anti-inflammatories, and even ibuprofen gel; however, her arthritis was really bothering her and did not seem to be much improved. I mixed some CBD oil in with a base cream of calendula, with some frankincense essential oil, and she also took some oral CBD capsules. Within a week, she was knitting again! Her family would often visit me to tell me how delighted they all were that she was able to knit again!

Another case was that of a sixty-six-year-old female patient who had been taking eight tramadol a day because she was suffering extreme pain with osteoarthritis, with her knees bothering her the most. She was heavily involved in the dog and horse worlds and very much wanted to walk her dogs, go to shows, and ride her horse, but the pain from the osteoarthritis had significantly impaired her ability to do any of this. She commenced a daily regimen of taking both a daytime and evening CBD product in addition to my usual turmeric, boswellia, trikatu formula. Within two months of commencing this routine, her pain was so significantly reduced that she was able to initially reduce (leaving the appropriate gap between it and the CBD), and finally give up all opioid pain relieving medication and merely indulged, in her own words, in the occasional "medicinal gin and tonic". She told me she didn't believe in miracles, but her pain was so significantly improved that she had been able to walk her dogs once more and participate in activities that had been impossible for so long that she was now convinced that her "herbal regimen" was her saviour.

Behçet's disease

Behçet's disease, or Behçet's syndrome, is a rare condition, which is difficult to diagnose as it has such a wide range of generalised symptoms but consists of inflammation of the blood vessels and tissues. Symptoms include genital and mouth ulcers, painful red eyes and blurred vision, acne, headaches, and painful, stiff, and swollen joints. In severe cases there are also risks of serious and potentially life-threatening issues such as permanent vision loss or strokes. The condition is subject to episodic flare-ups and relapses and also periods of remission.

I have had a patient who suffered from this condition and sadly she was one of those who had a stroke some twenty years ago as a very young woman. Her child at the time was only four years old, and she completely lost the power of speech and was paralysed, unable to walk, significantly impacting on her life and her ability to care for her child. Over the past twenty years she has relearnt speech, which is nevertheless slurred, and she has relearnt to walk, although she walks with a stick and struggles as one side is weaker than the other. In particular she struggles with pain while walking, negotiating stairs, and sleep issues. Since taking the CBD product, she has been able to reduce her pharmaceutical meds and described the effects to me as "magic". She had been using the product that was legal in Guernsey but not in the UK, with a slightly higher THC ratio than has thitherto been allowed in the UK. Her product contained 0.09% THC (rather than the UK 0.02%). Recently, she had run out for a while, and had to use a weaker product that she happened to have at home and discovered this did not work as well at controlling her symptoms as the slightly higher THC product, even though the amount of CBD in both products was identical.

Collagen connective tissue disorders

Collagen connective tissue disorders have become more researched and prevalent in the last twenty to thirty years, and encompass a variety of conditions such as Marfan syndrome, joint hypermobility syndrome, and also Ehlers-Danlos syndromes. Ehlers-Danlos syndromes are a hereditary group of connective tissue disorders that vary dramatically from sufferer to sufferer in both how they are affected by this and the genetic cause. The characteristics are usually joint hypermobility or joints that stretch further than normal (double jointed) and skin hyperextensibility (skin that can be stretched further than normal) and tissue fragility. There are many different subtypes which have different sets of clinical criteria to help diagnose. Confirmation is often by blood testing to establish which subtype the sufferer has. The most common is hypermobile EDS (hEDS). The symptoms include loose, unstable joints prone to dislocation and/or subluxation, joint pains, hyper-extendible joints, and early onset of osteoarthritis. Sufferers also have soft velvety like skin, which is sometimes more stretchy than in normal people, fragile skin that tears or bruises easily, scarring, slow and poor wound healing, and the development of molluscoid pseudo tumours (fleshy lesions associated with scars over pressure areas). There is also chronic, early onset debilitating musculoskeletal pain; there can be arterial, intestinal, and uterine fragility or rupture, scoliosis from birth and scleral fragility, poor muscle tone, mitral valve prolapse, and gum disease.

Each different type of the condition has a slightly different variation of connective tissue disorder. As connective tissue is what the body uses for strength and elasticity. This is a structural problem and can lead to lifelong pain and problems for its sufferers.

As a sufferer of Ehlers-Danlos syndrome myself, this is something I really understand. One becomes almost used to the regular dislocation and subluxation of joints, although one never becomes used to the pain—it is said that sufferers develop a higher pain tolerance than normal people because one regularly has to relocate joints that have subluxated or dislocated. I and both my daughters have this condition, and it has caused far-reaching issues with all of us. My younger daughter suffered a spinal cord injury after falling and her spine flexed, but the spinal cord did not, and nerves became trapped. More on this follows under the heading "Spinal cord injury" below;

however, in order to "treat" and live with this condition we have all been using CBD. I have been using turmeric capsules for around five years and then added CBD into the mix in around 2017. The difference in my ability to move, the reduction in pain on walking up and down stairs has been remarkable. In "the olden days" before I discovered herbal medicine, I would have to regularly have osteopathy, acupuncture, and sports massage. I now manage with far fewer outside therapies, and only the occasional massage or Bowen therapy in addition to my regular intake of CBD. Interestingly, this is meant to be a relatively rare condition, but I saw an unusually high number of patients with this condition in Guernsey. I could never quite work out why there was such a high proportion of EDS sufferers in such a small community—although as an aside, the number of dogs with epilepsy was also extremely high, and I often wondered whether it was something to do with the water (which is desalinated and very chemical) or the fact that the whole island is granite. I believe that the reason they came to see me was that they were all, like me, at the end of the road when it comes to what to use to manage the pain and inflammation in the body. And so they ended up coming to see me—herbalists are so often the "last hope" for many people. The combination of CBD with turmeric and often a CBD infused cream to apply topically has proved incredibly helpful for me and my patients alike.

COPD

Chronic obstructive pulmonary disease, otherwise known as COPD, is the name given to a group of conditions which are progressive and inflammatory, affecting the air flow to the lungs and making it difficult to breathe.

COPD is a term that covers a variety of different types of lung damage, the most common of which are chronic bronchitis, which is when the small airways (bronchioles) of the lung become narrower and inflamed, and emphysema, which is where the tiny air sacs (alveoli) at the end of the airways become damaged and irreversibly degenerated. The damage caused by COPD makes it more difficult for a person to take in air and thus harder to breathe. The airways lose their elasticity and can also make more mucus than is usual, which causes clogging.

Most commonly COPD is a direct result of cigarette smoking or exposure to irritating inhaled substances; dust, smoke, and air pollution can all cause problems. This is a slowly developing condition, its symptoms becoming more severe over time until it is almost impossible to perform even simple activities such as walking or cooking.

Symptomatically sufferers will often cough up a lot of mucus, suffer from shortness of breath, wheezing, and chest tightness. The symptoms often don't appear until there is already significant damage to the lungs, and this is a major cause of disability. COPD generally does not manifest until people are middle-aged or older. Having COPD increases the risk of respiratory infections, heart conditions, lung cancer, high blood pressure, as well as depression. COPD is irreversible and there is currently no cure for it. Treatment is predominantly symptomatic with inhalers, bronchodilators, and steroids.

As CBD is anti-inflammatory there is good potential for CBD to be helpful with COPD to help reduce the inflammation of the airways. Several terpenes such as caryophyllene, pinene, and linalool are also indicated in alleviating symptoms of asthma and breathing difficulties, so a CBD product rich in these terpenes would be ideal for the sufferer. Some of the cannabinoids found within cannabis have also been found to have bronchodilatory effects, thereby decreasing resistance in the respiratory airway and increasing air flow to the lungs. Cannabis activates the receptors CB-1 and CB-2 thus reducing airway inflammation.

Several of my patients and customers have suffered from chronic bronchitis and COPD and several with lung cancer, all of whom noticed significant improvement in their ease of breathing.

Epilepsy

Epilepsy is possibly the "one condition" that is currently hitting the news the most; and videos abound of children having seizures and being given a cannabis oil, and the seizures ending. There are a great many different types of epilepsy, but as previously mentioned cannabis as a medicine became considered a viable option after the publicity surrounding Charlotte Figi, the child with Dravet syndrome, and the production of Charlotte's Web CBD products. In the UK there have been several high-profile epilepsy cases, and these have caused a change in the law whereby it is now legal to prescribe high strength cannabis medicine in certain cases. Even so, this is rare, and not many doctors are qualified or trained to be able to prescribe, and the private prescription costs are prohibitive with costs as high as £900 a month being reported.

Whilst an "off the shelf" CBD product may not be quite as effective as the far stronger prescription types of cannabis medicine; I have still seen significant improvements with my customers and patients who have suffered from seizures. Generally, I would recommend an indica type product for such patients as the thinking is that a sativa product stimulates the brain too much, and because seizures are caused by a hyperexcitable neuronal network, further stimulating the network with a product that enhances brain activity is not recommended. It is not just *people* with seizures that we have found have significantly improved. We have seen major improvements in dogs, with customers willing to try anything to prevent their pet from having such seizures.

Fibromyalgia and polymyalgia rheumatica

This is the third most common condition that I see among patients. Fibromyalgia derived from the Latin *fibro* (for fibrous tissue) and *myalgia* which literally means pain in the muscles. Strongly related is polymyalgia also derived from the Latin *poly* (meaning many or diverse), thus the name means "diverse pain in the muscles".

These conditions are becoming more and more common in the twenty-first century. It has been mooted that endocannabinoid deficiency or dysregulation is the cause for an upsurge in autoimmune conditions. The sufferer has profound fatigue, and chronic and widespread pain—it has been reported to me that a patient may not even be touched gently without feeling pain; there is also the famous "fibro-fog"—lack of clarity of thinking, memory loss, and forgetfulness. The patient suffers pain everywhere, sometimes worst in the hips, knees, and shoulders, those areas that are most used, and it can sometimes be worse than others: when it is particularly bad this is known as a "fibro flare". Often these patients are completely exhausted, and many have days when they cannot get out of bed, completely drained of all energy.

These patients suffer extreme pain and no matter how many tests they undergo, no cause can be found. With fibromyalgia there is now a test performed by general practitioners which involves establishing if the pain has been present for three months or more, with the focus on eighteen points on the body where if pressed the patient feels excruciating pain. These tender spots are usually not noticed by the patient unless they are pressed. Other associated conditions alongside the muscular aches and pains include the inability to sleep well, waking up in pain, headaches, and irritable bowel syndrome with alternating diarrhoea or constipation; this can be accompanied by bloating or nausea, lack of concentration, dizziness, clumsiness, and sensitivity to weather changes, noise, smoke, lights, and other environmental factors.

There is no known cause, although anecdotally a lot of these patients have had some form of trigger such as glandular fever as a child, a fall, a traumatic event, but often this condition manifests without any obvious trigger.

Pharmaceutically this condition is often treated with steroids, pain relievers, NSAIDs, opiates, pregabalin, gabapentin, amitriptyline, antidepressants, muscle relaxants, and sleeping pills. Many of these have significant side effects and many patients report feeling "spaced out" or discombobulated by these medications.

In practice I have seen hundreds of fibromyalgia patients—they are probably about equal to the number of arthritis patients I see, in a predominantly elder community, but I see this condition in young people as well as the elderly.

These patients often benefit from a two pronged regime, whereby they take two different types of CBD, one that contains more beta-caryophyllene and myrcene for the night-time to allow for an improved sleep pattern and one that is richer in limonene and pinene during the daytime, which will improve their mental clarity and elevate their mood. Both types will be a reasonable strength of CBD to give the anti-inflammatory effects. In addition, of course, I would always prescribe my turmeric, boswellia, and trikatu capsules.

PCOS

Polycystic ovarian syndrome or polycystic ovarian disease is often abbreviated to PCOS. This is a condition affecting females of any age and is resultant from a hormonal imbalance. Predominantly caused by an excess in testosterone in women, its physical signs include acne, weight gain, hirsutism, and male pattern baldness as well as amenorrhoea (absence of menstruation), dysmenorrhoea (painful menstruation), abnormally heavy flow, pelvic pain, thickening of the uterine wall and, as indicated by its name, multiple cysts upon the ovaries. The menstrual irregularity causes fertility issues, and ovaries may also develop several fluid collections which prevent the regular release of eggs. When one endocrine system is imbalanced, this often causes imbalance in the entire endocrine system and can thus cause an increase in insulin and a concomitant thyroid imbalance. A regular imbalance in insulin can obviously also risk the development of type 2 diabetes.

Along with hormonal imbalance come mood swings and the likelihood of developing depression, low mood, and stress-related conditions.

As a homeostatic regulator, CBD is a potential good option for this condition as it can help to balance out the entire endocrine system and ensure that menstrual regularity is regained. However, as CBD is also mood-elevating and calming, this can also help the patient with low mood and mild depression.

PMDD/PMS

Premenstrual dysphoric disorder (PMDD) is an extremely severe form of premenstrual syndrome which causes many emotional and physical symptoms monthly in the week or two before a period commences. Many people suffer from mild symptoms of PMS, but with PMDD these symptoms can be significantly worse, to such an extent that the person suffering from this condition may find it difficult to work, to socialise, to have healthy relationships, and in extreme cases this can even lead to suicidal thoughts.

The emotional symptoms of PMDD can include the likes of mood swings, and feeling upset, angry, irritable, anxious, hopeless, overwhelmed, tense, and on edge. Also, difficulty concentrating, lack of energy, and a complete disinterest in activities normally enjoyed. Physically the symptoms include such things as breast pain, tenderness, or swelling, muscular or joint pains, headaches, a bloated feeling, appetite changes, sleep problems, and a host of others.

CBD works very well as an anti-inflammatory and thus muscle relaxant, aiding with period cramps, gut and bowel cramps, and similar aches and pains. As a pain management device CBD has been shown to have significant benefits in this regard, and for those suffering who experience mood swings, there is a sense of calm, an easing of anxiety and depression.

Irritable bowel, ulcerative colitis, and other gastrointestinal conditions

As discussed previously we now know that we have cannabinoid receptors (CB-1 and CB-2) in every organ system of the human body creating the endocannabinoid system. This helps to modulate the endocrine system, supports immunological responses, and controls inflammation within the body. Evidence is growing to show that the endocannabinoid system is particularly heavily involved in many processes of the gastrointestinal system, which includes the cellular growth of the gut lining, pain perception, and gut and bowel motility amongst others. We have vast quantities of cannabinoid receptors in the gastrointestinal system, so it does stand to reason that the ingestion of a CBD product could alleviate many gastrointestinal conditions. In addition, a great many gut and bowel disorders stem from an increase in anxiety or stress, both of which can cause irritable bowel, constipation, or diarrhoea. Again, as CBD has been shown to alleviate anxiety and promote stress resilience this also points to a holistic approach of alleviating one condition and thereby reducing the symptoms it causes. By supporting a healthy inflammatory response with the ingestion of a CBD product gastrointestinal conditions can be markedly improved.

I have many patients with irritable bowel syndrome and several with ulcerative colitis. One man in particular had been suffering from ulcerative colitis for many years. This was a debilitating condition for him, and he often had to take time off work when he was having what he called an "episode". Since taking the CBD along with some slippery elm and turmeric, this man has not had a single day off work owing to illness. Interestingly, he was away for a few weeks, and ran out of his CBD halfway through his holiday. There was no immediate reaction, his symptoms did not return for some time, but after he returned from leave, he popped in to see me and having not had CBD for around ten days at that point, said the symptoms were beginning to return. He was quick to start his CBD regime again, and the next time I saw him, all symptoms were again in remission. This once again is an indication that CBD only seems to work while the person is taking it: it does not cure conditions, but ameliorates their effects.

Menopause

As a woman ages, so her levels of oestrogen and progesterone decline to the point where menstruation ceases. Although the adrenal glands begin to attempt to compensate for this reduction in sex hormones by producing hormones to deal with the imbalance, this can cause issues and adrenal fatigue becomes a problem. These issues also occur after a hysterectomy.

Symptoms, well known to millions of women worldwide, are fatigue, hot flushes, low libido, vaginal dryness, night sweats, mood swings, midlife crisis, depression, and insomnia. Associated conditions with the hormonal imbalance are also loss of bone density (osteoporosis) and heart and arterial disease.

Prior to the menopause starting fully, there is a period of several years called "perimenopause", and often this entire indisposition can last many years from anywhere in the early to mid-forties up until the early sixties.

Research has found that endocannabinoids act as a major neuromodulatory system in various physiological and behavioural functions, being regulated in part by gonadal hormones. Receptors and metabolic enzymes of the endocannabinoid system are predominantly located on structures within the hypothalamic–pituitary–gonadal axis. It has been posited that changes in the levels of sex hormones alter the way the endocannabinoid system signals. Research is showing that there are significant changes in the endocannabinoid system during menopausal transition. As oestrogen facilitates proper endocannabinoid system function by regulating fatty acid amide hydrolase (FAAH) levels in the blood, when the production of oestrogen in the body declines, this causes a drop in FAAH levels, thereby creating an imbalance. Additionally, the endocannabinoid, anandamide, also has an ovarian function as it aids in the maturation and release of the egg during ovulation. Oestrogen activates the endocannabinoid system for the regulation of emotional response. The declining interactions between the endocannabinoid system and oestrogen lead to the theory that menopausal symptoms may arise from a reduction in endocannabinoid activity.

To balance the endocannabinoid system with the use of CBD should ameliorate some of the effects of the menopause. For example, osteoporosis—loss of bone density—can occur during the menopause. Because oestrogen levels are declining, and oestrogen regulates bone cell growth, there is a high risk of menopausal women developing osteoporosis. Research has indicated that CBD can interact with receptors to prevent bone density loss.

One of the most frustrating and common side effects of the menopause is hot flushes. Anandamide helps in the regulation of body temperature and as CBD increases the levels of anandamide in the body by inhibiting the action of FAAH this can help the body to self-regulate body temperature more effectively.

Menopausal women often suffer from insomnia, which may well exacerbate the other symptoms including low mood. Long-term insomnia will seriously impact on mood and other areas of life. CBD has been shown to be remarkably effective at helping promote a healthy sleep pattern and is also anxiolytic which is an additional benefit for a menopausal woman.

The menopause can also elicit painful conditions in the sufferer, including generalised aches and pains, stiff joints, and migraines. Research has indicated that CBD can be a highly effective aid in pain management. Its anti-inflammatory action will help all aspects of this tiresome condition.

As the hormonal balance in the perimenopausal and menopausal woman fluctuates her mood will equally fluctuate and this can often be accompanied by anxiety. Stressful life changes manifest as anxiety, fatigue, and pain, and again this is where CBD could be incredibly helpful.

Many patients report all of these symptoms described above and more when they come to see me with menopausal issues, and in almost every case (apart from one, I believe, who wanted an increase in her libido and found it was, in her case, not significantly improved) there has been significant improvement in all the symptoms listed.

Migraines

Migraine headaches are a very common condition with countless sufferers reported worldwide. A mild headache can escalate to something far more severe and pounding, with nausea, vomiting, light sensitivity, and auditory or visual disturbance. I have seen significant success with migraine headaches in practice. One particular patient came after having three days off work weekly for the previous few weeks as her migraines were now cyclical and happening almost every few days, which was completely debilitating. She had changed her diet, excluded all known triggers, and really was at her wit's end.

A huge issue for her was the vomiting and nausea that accompanied her headaches. We started her on an extremely low dose of CBD initially to see if there was any reaction. A few days later she came back to see me, and reported this had helped to dull the symptoms significantly. She stayed on the low dose for around a month before increasing her dose very slightly. This was an ongoing patient whom I saw very regularly and she enjoyed an almost complete remission of her symptoms, with only a few mild headaches reported since starting on a regime of CBD. As mentioned previously, my daughter has suffered from debilitating migraines since she was a small child, and she has also found significant benefit from using CBD oil, topically as well as ingested. By rubbing some cream containing CBD oil together with some lavender essential oil, which is also considered useful for migraine headaches, we are able to control and reduce her headaches considerably.

Multiple sclerosis

Multiple sclerosis is a fairly common autoimmune inflammatory disease that affects the brain and spinal cord, causing a variety of issues, including visual disturbance, and problems with limb movement, sensation, and balance. The immune system attacks the myelin sheath, which covers the neurons of the brain and spinal cord, and this interferes with the functional ability of the nerves. It is a lifelong condition that can cause severe disability. It is one of the most common causes of disability in young adults. There have been many studies performed on the ability of cannabis to treat multiple sclerosis, and cannabis-based drug Sativex, manufactured by GW Pharmaceuticals, is specifically targeted at MS sufferers. Sativex has been shown to be effective for spasticity, peripheral neuropathy, and pain.

Symptoms of multiple sclerosis include fatigue, difficulty walking, visual problems including blurred vision, issues with bladder control, numbness or tingling in different body parts, muscle stiffness and spasms, issues with coordination and balance, and cognitive impairment affecting thinking, planning, or learning.

On one occasion a woman was brought to see me by her extremely concerned son. She was suffering from multiple sclerosis and was having an "episode". She told me that when she has these "episodes" sometimes her lungs simply do not want to work and feel like they are collapsing, meaning she struggles to breathe and cannot talk. She arrived heavily supported by her son, who virtually had to carry her out of the car, and we had to organise a seat for her within the shop itself, so she could rest, as she lacked the ability to stand for any length of time. During the discussion she was given a sample of a 60% CBD paste with a slightly higher level of THC than is currently legally allowed in the UK but is legally viable in Guernsey. Several people aided her son getting her back into the car, as she was very stiff, and struggling to get back in.

The following day another woman came into the shop telling us she had seen a miracle. Her sister (the MS sufferer) had apparently telephoned her as she reached home, some twenty minutes after being in the shop. Not only did this woman get out of the car unaided and walk to her house, she then telephoned her sister and spent half an hour on the telephone with her. As mentioned in the previous paragraph, when she first came to see me, her lungs were feeling "irritated and like they were collapsing"—precluding her from speaking. For her to then walk unaided to her house, and be able to hold a telephone conversation such a brief time after being so debilitated, was nothing short of a miracle—according to the patient.

The customer's sister was so impressed she came in to stock up on products to replicate this twenty-minute complete remission of symptoms! There were many success stories in a similar vein with local customers suffering from neurodegenerative conditions.

Skin conditions

Cannabinoid receptors, both CB-1 and CB-2 are found throughout the integumentary system (skin). It is thought that the endocannabinoid system regulates cell growth and wound healing and it also plays a huge part in immunological response and thus could be significantly helpful in the treatment of inflammatory skin conditions. Anti-tumour effects are also reasonably well documented with skin cancers showing significant improvements with the application of a CBD rich balm.

Many of my patients use CBD rich creams and balms for a variety of skin conditions including eczema, psoriasis, sun damage, pruritis, and folliculitis. In addition, we are seeing good results with the ingestion of an oil or capsule—because ultimately, skin conditions come from an imbalance within.

Sleep

Poor and disrupted sleep has wide-reaching effects upon a person's quality of life. It is also implicated in a lot of conditions, which cause lack of sleep—and there is the circular argument that lack of sleep causes or exacerbates certain conditions such as anxiety or stress.

Almost all my patients using CBD for a variety of conditions report that they are able to sleep better since using the product. Invariably, I will give these patients a capsule as it appears to have a longer half-life in the body so that they stay asleep throughout the night instead of waking at 3 am and lie tossing and turning with revolving thoughts. For sleep I would always recommend the more soporific indica strain of product, something that is rich in linalool and myrcene which are the relaxing terpenes.

Spinal cord injury

I have first-hand experience of this condition. In February 2017, my daughter fell in a health spa, and hit her coccyx on the floor and her head against a wall. Within a few hours she had lost feeling in her feet, which gradually spread up her body until she lost bladder control and then went higher. Approximately from mid-waist (T-10 on the thoracic spine) downwards she had no feeling whatsoever. I explained to the wonderful staff at the hospital that my daughter had a collagen connective tissue disorder; however, they initially felt that this could not be the cause of the paraplegia. After eight weeks on a geriatric ward and no progress being made, she was moved to orthopaedics, where for several more weeks no progress was made. She was on a cocktail of morphine, gabapentin, laxatives, and other painkillers. There was no change in her condition whatsoever. Finally, after around four months she was moved to a neurological rehabilitation ward. Eventually, having exhausted the hospital orthopaedics and house neurologists, a neurologist arrived who understood Ehlers-Danlos syndrome and how that can work—her spine flexed when she fell but her spinal cord did not. This resulted in pinched nerves and the loss of feeling she had in her lower limbs. In frustration, I had written to the hospital and asked if I could treat her myself and was given permission. I brought in several other therapists, my friend a homeopath and craniosacral practitioner, a Bowen therapist, a sports massage therapist, to assist me, a medical herbalist. Between us, we commenced a regime of treatments, consisting of a homeopathic remedy, turmeric capsules, St. John's wort oil topically applied, and CBD capsules. The combination of therapies and supplements got her out of that hospital in under a month from the beginning of our treatment of her—even though they had said she would be in neurorehab for months, possibly up to a year and that after two years she would be the "best she'll ever be". She came home on crutches and commenced taking the CBD daily. One year later, she travelled to Guernsey to help me out in the shop. She is still not fully recovered and may never recover full function and feeling in her legs, but she feels that CBD certainly helped with her pain levels, her ability to sleep, the inflammation, and also with her mood and energy levels.

Sciatica and piriformis syndrome

Piriformis syndrome is a troublesome and painful condition caused by aggravation or pressure on the sciatic nerve close to the piriformis muscle. The piriformis muscle sits under the gluteus maximus connecting the lowest spinal vertebrae with the upper part of the leg. The sciatic nerve runs through a space in the pelvic bone and the nerve and muscle are adjacent to each other; hence the troublesome issues should there be any inflammation or muscular spasm in this area. In many cases when people think they have sciatica, they are in fact suffering from piriformis syndrome.

People suffering from piriformis syndrome will often complain of sciatica, or a sharp radiating pain from the buttock or lower back down the leg and into the thigh, calf, and foot. Additionally, the person will have difficulty in sitting or putting weight on their buttock on one side; they will have a muscular spasm within the piriformis muscle itself and also pain in the piriformis muscle during a rectal examination. Sciatica type pain ensues when the hip is moved and rotated against resistance.

The causes can be manifold, but many cases come from sitting for too long and can also include conditions such as abnormal development of the piriformis muscle or sciatic nerve. Other causes of piriformis syndrome could be scoliosis, unusually vigorous exercises, underlying medical conditions, foot conditions, leg length discrepancy, and also certain hip conditions or prior to hip surgery. Often the cause is difficult to identify. The underlying condition is one of pain and inflammation. CBD is anti-inflammatory and pain relieving, so this is ideal to use in conditions such as these.

CHAPTER 16

CBD as a daily general health supplement

Having run several health stores, and one that specialises in cannabis extract supplements, I have now seen thousands of patients and customers who are benefitting from the daily ingestion of cannabis extracts. Many people who have no specific condition other than "life"—that is, generally feeling a little bit stressed, sometimes a little fatigued but who also want a health supplement they can take daily with no negative side effects but which may help to balance their bodies—are turning to CBD as a potential supplement.

I genuinely feel that having this supplement has changed the lives of so many people that I have seen. They report feeling generally more energised, they tell me they are finally sleeping through the night, they have less pain, and less brain fog. Many of my customers take the supplement as a general "well-being" thing, the same as you might take vitamin B complex or vitamin C supplements, and often it transpires, in the hopes of warding off anything more serious that might hit them in years to come.

CBD for athletes

Many athletes are used to pushing themselves to the limit to overcome all the intense physical demands that are part of their sport and their continual challenge. It is therefore unsurprising that pain and injuries are extremely common amongst athletes from all sports, and in an effort to achieve, to win, and to push themselves, athletes often overlook potential risks and health concerns. This can lead to long-term conditions and health issues.

It is possible that CBD could potentially be an amazing tool for athletes from all sports to deliver a wide range of benefits and therapeutic properties. CBD can help with pain management, muscle recovery, stress relief, and mood regulation.

Athletes are continually pushing themselves to the limits, which of course, will result in occasional injuries and aches and pains. Often, they will resort to over the counter painkillers such as ibuprofen or paracetamol, but this is not without risk. Research has shown that long-term use of such over the counter medicines can cause liver damage, increase the risk of strokes, heart attacks, gastric disturbance and bleeding, and a variety of other health conditions.

Because CBD is an anti-inflammatory agent, it can significantly reduce the swelling and pain caused by inflammation. CBD influences the TPRV1 vanilloid receptors which mediate pain perception.

CBD is also full of flavonoids which are antioxidants and some consider the antioxidant potential of CBD to be more powerful than vitamin C or vitamin D. Reducing oxidative stress and aiding recovery for an athlete could make CBD a really valuable option.

Stress and anxiety, for example the pre-game or match stress, can also be significantly improved and alleviated with the use of CBD. Another issue for many athletes is sleep. It is important to get enough sleep to enable recovery and to ensure no restlessness; again this is something CBD is particularly good at.

Is it possible for a professional athlete to use CBD?

Many sports organisations do not allow athletes to consume certain substances and this has brought into question, historically, even substances like salbutamol, in an asthma inhaler, which can "speed up" the heart rate and be considered "inadmissible". With a substance so closely related to THC, the substance that "makes people high", it is understandable that many sports organisations will be conflicted. However, the times are changing and many are beginning to recognise CBD for its therapeutic properties and potential, and are permitting its use, although there are still some organisations that have enforced policies strictly prohibiting athletes from using CBD.

The benefits offered to an athlete from the regular use of CBD include:

- Energy
- Relief from muscular and joint pain
- A more balanced system
- Improved breathing
- Better recovery after sport
- Reduction of anxiety before events
- General wellness.

Information regarding COVID-19—the coronavirus

2020 has been the year of the coronavirus—which cannot have passed anyone by. Initially there was much discussion around the fact that CBD being immunomodulatory might not be a good thing to take at this time, but exciting new research has shown that it could in fact be ideal.

Researchers from the Medical College and Dental Colleges of Georgia in the USA have reported laboratory experimentation showing CBD's ability to improve oxygen levels and reduce inflammation and lung damage from adult respiratory distress syndrome (ARDS). CBD appears to reduce the cytokine storm that damages the lungs. The study discusses that the levels of the peptide apelin reduce with the viral infection; however, CBD can quickly normalise these levels along with lung function. Their dramatic research evidenced the shifting of the peptide apelin levels in both circulating blood and lung tissue. Blood levels of the peptide dropped near to zero in their model and increased twenty-fold with CBD, it is claimed in the *Journal of Cellular and Molecular Medicine*.

Apelin is a widespread peptide manufactured with the blood, lung, heart, brain, and fat tissue, and is a regulatory factor in reducing both blood pressure and inflammation. When a patient's blood pressure rises, apelin levels would normally rise in order to bring it down. However, during the study it was found that with the coronavirus infection, apelin neither rose nor brought blood pressure down but instead decreased in both lung tissue and circulation, until CBD was administered. The researchers found that CBD enabled improvements in lung function, healthier oxygen levels, and repair of some of the structural damage to the lungs. The study concluded that more work was needed, including human trials before it should be recommended as part of a treatment plan for COVID-19. Further research is ongoing to better understand the interaction between CBD, apelin, and the coronavirus. It is suspected that the virus suppresses apelin in some way, and that CBD interacts with this; however, the researchers feel that there are likely other benefits to use of CBD.

During the study the researchers found that treatment with CBD normalised the immune response of the subjects as well as their apelin and oxygen levels, at the same time regulating the scarring in the lungs characteristic of ARDS.

The apelinergic system is ubiquitous according to Jack Yu, one of the researchers. He explains that apelin does diverse jobs throughout the body and that levels may rise and fall; however, levels are consistently measurable in the lungs, making it a good biomarker.

Synthetic agonists that increase apelin are showing promise in the laboratory for cardiovascular disease, including slowing the growth rate of weak points in blood vessels (aneurysms). The researchers concluded that CBD appeared to be a natural apelin agonist. This could be very exciting for the future of CBD with a variety of conditions and may explain why in practice it appears to be helpful for so many situations.

An article by Esposito et al., in the *British Journal of Pharmacology* of July 2020, calls for more targeted studies to test cannabidiol as a support drug against the COVID-19 pandemic. The authors posit that cannabis extracts may down-regulate the expression of two key receptors for SARS-CoV2 in models of human epithelia. They also suggest that as cannabidiol has such a wide range of immunomodulatory and anti-inflammatory effects it could mitigate uncontrolled cytokine production which is responsible for lung injury. This concept is borne out by the research of the Georgia team. Esposito's team suggest that as cannabidiol is a peroxisome proliferator-activated receptor agonist (PPARy) that it could display "direct antiviral activity" and "regulation of fibroblast/myofibroblast activation and inhibition of the development of pulmonary fibrosis" which they suggest would ameliorate lung function in recovered patients.

Long COVID

It is estimated by the National Institute for Health Research that at the time of writing (November 2020) at least 60,000 people in the UK are suffering the effects of so-called "long COVID" which have only recently been defined by UK health bodies, the National Institute for Health and Care Excellence (NICE), the Scottish Intercollegiate Guidelines Network (SIGN), and the Royal College of GPs (RCGP), who in October 2020 defined "long COVID" as follows:

> Signs and symptoms that develop during or following an infection consistent with COVID-19, continue for more than 12 weeks and are not explained by an alternative diagnosis. It usually presents with clusters of symptoms,

often overlapping, which can fluctuate and change over time and can affect any system in the body.

Post-COVID-19 syndrome may be considered before 12 weeks while the possibility of an alternative underlying disease is also being assessed.

The document lists the following signs and symptoms that can affect different body systems, and can overlap and change over time, including *"cardiovascular, respiratory, gastrointestinal, neurological, musculoskeletal, metabolic, renal, dermatological, otolaryngological, haematological, and autonomic systems. In addition, patients may have psychiatric problems, generalised pain, fatigue, and persistent fever."*

Full guidelines which are still to be published will cover pharmacological and non-pharmacological interventions as well as best practice for "long COVID" recovery and rehabilitation services. They anticipate that this will be a "living" guideline which will be subject to updates as these become available and new evidence is discovered.

CHAPTER 17

CBD in practice—a few testimonials and stories

In August 2018, I moved to Guernsey in the Channel Islands to manage a shop and herbal medicine practice, specialising in cannabis extracts and supplements.

The range of cannabis extracts on sale was extremely diverse and also included a wide range of herbal over the counter remedies.

Because the terpenes within the plant (as well as the flavonoids and cannaflavins) are so varied and can differ from plant to plant, which is why it's so hard to standardise a dose, we are seeing a variety of effects with patients.

In Guernsey, the law is slightly different to the UK and allows the use of a higher level of THC than is permitted in the UK. The ratio may be 3% THC to 100% CBD. As no plant would ever have 100% CBD unless it was an isolate this means that the highest amount of THC available was 1.8% in the 60% CBD "paste". This proved to have an incredible synergistic effect—the CBD and THC together seeming to work incredibly well on patients with MS, cancer, PTSD, and chronic pain.

On the first day of opening, a woman came into the shop in tears. Her father had just been diagnosed with inoperable lung cancer. The tumour was too large to remove and it had spread to his lymph nodes. She was utterly distraught! She was given the lowest of the oils we had in stock, which is a 3%

CBD—0.09% THC. After a week of taking up to three drops daily of this, we changed her father onto the 6% oil, which contains 0.18% THC. She came back to see us regularly to report on how her father was doing.

After three weeks, she came in to report that he'd had to travel to the mainland to the hospital to see the oncologist. Miraculously, the cancer was no longer present in the lymph: we were told that at the scan there was evidence something had been there, but nothing was showing up. Fast forward a few months and the man is told his tumour, initially inoperable, has now reduced in size and could be operable. His progress continues to improve, and at the very least his quality of life has improved without measure.

Fibromyalgia and cancer—testimonial

Here, in her own words, that particular customer tells her story.

> I am writing this testimonial, not only for myself, but for my stepfather who was diagnosed with lung cancer in August 2018. Both our lives would have a very different outcome if we did not have access to CBD oil. My testimonial and others will never be able to do justice to this natural product and make others appreciate the benefits until you are struck down by a cancer or a health condition which affects your ability to function on a daily basis.
>
> I am a 40-year-old female diagnosed Nov 2018 with fibromyalgia. This diagnosis came after a string of unfortunate events and with already established diagnosis of ME several years ago. In August 2018 I was diagnosed with a rare kidney infection that required seven days of intravenous antibiotics and fluids. As a result of this I had a miscarriage and also a severe reaction to the intravenous medication. The kidney infection is a strain which is immune to all oral antibiotics and the intravenous

medication was under instruction by a specialist microbiologist in Birmingham as there is no such specialist over in Guernsey.

Within this same week we were moving house, I was under pressure at work, receiving messages from 5.30 am, my son had severely dislocated his leg at school, my mum had collapsed needing another ambulance, and my dad was diagnosed with lung cancer. Needless to say, the extreme stress and anxiety was unbearable and resulted in a later diagnosis of fibromyalgia and further kidney infections requiring intravenous medication and specialist appointments and hospital stays.

I no longer work due to this and I have been on an array of medication which means I cannot drive when I'm taking them and leaves me confused and forgetful. The pain is unbearable and I have been referred to the rheumatology specialist since January 2019 but the only contact I have had is a letter from them stating there is a waiting list for appointments and they are unable to offer a date as yet but they are sending this letter as confirmation I am on the waiting list.

This condition along with ME and recurring kidney infections is extremely depressing especially when I was an active, outgoing, independent, busy person working 9-hour days. My life has drastically changed, I need assistance getting out of bed some mornings and doing basic daily tasks and various muscles go into spasm. I was no longer able to walk my dogs twice a day, unable to wash and dry my hair frequently, everything you take for granted.

Then I started taking CBD capsules, my spasms still occur but a lot less frequently in a day, and the swellings in my hands and feet have reduced. I can take my son to activities and school after taking the capsules which keep the pain at bay till I get home to take my strong painkillers. I can take my dogs on very short walks every other day, yes maybe not as often as I would like or as long as I like but the CBD has given me my independence back. I feel a lot more relaxed mentally, as all these conditions and life events had a huge impact on my mental health too, leaving me extremely depressed and I'm ashamed to say, suicidal. It has allowed me to regain my self-respect and feel human.

As to my Dad's diagnosis of lung cancer the CBD oil along with the paste has been phenomenal. My Dad is 71 and has had a stroke prior to his diagnosis. He was told it was a significantly large tumour and he, due to other medical complications, was unable to undergo surgery to remove the tumour. Also, on the specialist cancer scan there were a couple of lymph nodes showing cancer.

By luck, fate, whatever you wish to call it, I started straight away to read up on treatments and testimonials and studies done for alternative cancer treatments. I came to read the overwhelming amount of literature on CBD; I had learned of the herbal shop in the local press and I contacted the shop and straight away was given advice and told that this was not a cure and they did not wish to fill me with misleading information or false promises.

I bought CBD and went to my Dad and relayed everything I had learnt. My parents as myself are not open to drugs and I have brought my children up with zero tolerance so I was pleasantly surprised that he was willing to give it a go as he and my Mum are the older generation and stuck in their ways. The first amazing result was that his breathing greatly improved within a week. He was able to sleep and relax. The second was the next PET scan before treatment commenced and there were no active live cancer cells in his lymph nodes. This could not be explained.

He then went for seven weeks of intensive chemo and radiation treatment in Southampton. He was informed that he would lose his appetite and it was imperative he must eat and they would monitor his food intake and he would feel very nauseous, also irritated skin from the radiation.

Well, what a miracle, no sickness, never lost his appetite (actually gained weight), and only very slight burning. The only side effect from the treatment was that after a huge dose of chemo they give you high strength steroids and my Dad got extremely down and anxious and emotional. This was a very common side effect of the strong steroids and was quickly averted.

He has now been back since Christmas and been told the tumour has significantly reduced, exceeding expectations and is due next month for his final scan and evaluation.

"Yes!" I hear the sceptics say, "Yes, well, he has had chemo and radiotherapy, of course it would shrink," and yes, we have to give credit to this and it could very well have played a major role, but we can honestly put down to CBD the ease in breathing, keeping and gaining appetite, fewer burns, relaxing and loss of anxiety. My Dad not only had the stress of being diagnosed with a significant lung cancer tumour, but also added stress as a proper old Guernsey man, stuck in his ways and never going off-island who would prefer eating my Mum's meals than going out or being out of his comfort zone on so many levels and having multiple appointments and treatments in a very large hospital. CBD has played a huge role and we cannot recommend it enough. I have recommended CBD to anyone and everyone. Some at first think, "Oh yeah, I will try" it but never do; it's one of those fads. So, I give them several of my capsules and then they are converted. From friends with arthritis to a friend with a hiatus hernia, to depression, to a nan who lost so much weight and is now gaining. I am hopeful we will in the future be able to get it through prescription and the medical patches, as on the fibromyalgia research site this has had huge backing and recommendations and has transformed patients' lives dramatically.

But for now, I would hopefully be able to show and educate others to try CBD and prove it does change people's quality of life over a wide range of health complaints.

Anxiety and post cancer malaise

A fifty-two-year-old female patient came to see me, initially with anxiety and an inability to sleep. During the consultation it transpired she had historically also been suffering from pancreatitis, had just had a bilateral salpingo-oophorectomy, was suffering from diabetes, and had also been diagnosed less than a year previously with primary breast cancer which had metastasised into her bones. She had already received radiotherapy and a shoulder and humerus bone replacement. The patient was displaying an extremely low mood, was weepy, and explained that she was constantly anxious about life, about cancer, and felt like she had a "tight ball" in her stomach. She was feeling sick constantly. Her most recent blood test cancer markers had gone back up and she was at the end of her tether.

The patient complained that her energy levels were at least half of what they had been the previous year and was also suffering from night sweats which she felt were cold—she did not feel hot, rather cold, but still perspiring profusely. She brought a facecloth into the consultation with her, and had to mop at her forehead regularly during the consultation. She also complained that her gut was not right, and that she had a kind of "tension headache" almost constantly.

Initially, this patient was prescribed an herbal medicine tincture combination, and additionally some CBD products. Alongside that she was given a sleep syrup and an antioxidant mushroom complex.

She returned for her first follow-up with me two weeks later, and already by this point she was feeling much brighter in herself. Her negative feelings and sad thoughts had become far less problematic and she had even started going to the gym and swimming during the previous week. She felt that her gut was significantly improved.

One month further on she felt that her anxiety levels had rescinded completely but that her night sweats were now increased. Throughout the first six weeks I kept the patient on the same herbal regime as well as her CBD capsules. I slightly changed her herbal prescription for the following month and she returned with her blood test results. Remarkably cancer markers were now within normal limits and everything apart from one of her liver function tests had now normalised. Her oncologist was amazed and very pleased with her progress.

During the third month, she came to see me with the epithet. "I feel fantastic." Her bloods were normalising further, the liver function test that was very slightly off in the previous month had improved again, and she told me she "doesn't think about cancer any more".

Two months later, the patient's blood test results were all within normal parameters and her emotional state was balanced and she felt "great". Throughout, and on an ongoing basis, this patient has taken a CBD capsule for the daytime, one for the night-time, and her supplements. Two years on, this patient still receives her herbal tincture regularly from me and is convinced that this and her CBD is the thing that is keeping her blood tests at normal levels, and is so afraid of feeling how she "used to" that she says she will be staying on this regime for the foreseeable future.

Severe mental health concerns

A female fifty-seven-year-old patient with significant mental health issues came to see me. This poor woman had been feeling suicidal and had made several attempts upon her life.

She had been prescribed a smorgasbord of pharmaceuticals in an attempt to balance and normalise her. Her mental state was incredibly fragile. She wept several times throughout the consultation and it transpired that she had been abused as a child, had been in an abusive relationship, and had been through several incredibly traumatic life incidents, one involving a shop robbery where a gun was pointed at her and others which I feel would be improper to share here. Significant trauma.

Throughout life terrible things seemed to have happened to her, impacting on her relationships with her husband(s) and children. She was at her wit's end. I prescribed an herbal prescription and some CBD to support her. She had been suffering panic attacks and pain in her solar plexus similar to nausea, but a pressing pain. Sleep was an issue. Within three weeks of commencing the regime of CBD and the herbal mixture, this patient was telling me she felt "normal" for the first time in years. This was punctuated by her partner telephoning me to tell me that this was the best he'd seen her in a very long time. This patient remains on regular doses of CBD both during the day and night to help her get through her emotional difficulties and to aid with sleep. She feels like a new woman.

Chronic regional pain syndrome—testimonial

This is a story written by a colleague and friend about her son and how CBD has changed his life. This was written over a year ago, and in the interim year this lad has improved even further.

> In only 12 short months my boy has taken back control of his life and is now living it to the max!
>
> One year ago tonight I gave him two drops of CBD oil after three months of chronic and prolonged illness had completely incapacitated him. He had vomited almost every day from January to March and we were

all despairing because his quality of life was so poor, he had lost so much weight and his body was wracked with agonising neurological pain which we couldn't even treat with the horrible cocktail of naproxen, gabapentin and amitriptyline he had been taking since he was 5 years old because he simply couldn't keep anything in his stomach.

G has CRPS, cyclical vomiting syndrome, Raynaud's, hypermobility in his major joints and hypomobility of his spine. He has life-threatening allergies and has food intolerances. He took a combination of 14 prescription medications which were arguably far more dangerous to my boy than the dreadful medical conditions they were supposed to treat. His mood was low, his brain "foggy" and he had developed OCD tendencies. He never slept right through as he needed pain relief top-ups despite wearing lidocaine patches. We were living day by day and G wasn't even able to practise his beloved archery—he just wasn't strong enough.

Fast forward 12 months ...

- No longer taking any prescription meds except antihistamine.
- Replaced all the pain meds with CBD water soluble, capsules, oil and CBD balm.
- Introduced turmeric, black pepper, l-carnitine, Q10, D3, omega fish oils, magnesium and B12.
- Increased schooling from 55—92%.
- Grown 6 inches, gained weight and feet jumped three sizes.
- Started his archery training again.
- Won four Scottish titles and a UK & Ireland championship.
- Started sleeping through the night and hasn't stopped.
- Has changed completely in mood and spirit. He's laughing and joking again describing his life now as having had the brightness dialled up to max.

As G's mum I cannot begin to describe how amazed and delighted I am with the changes in G. He has never looked so well; his colour is great and he has so much more energy. His renewed enthusiasm for life is as fabulous as his story inspirational.

His medical conditions may be lifelong but they no longer define him and whilst he'll never be "cured" he now has a quality of life we could only have imagined before CBD.

(Words used with kind permission from Mrs B., Harrow)

Polypharmacy and pain

A twenty-five-year-old female patient, a mother of three, was taking a combination of gapapentin, oramorph, diclofenac, and zapain (co-codamol) for a condition arising from herniated discs and nerve impingement in her spine. She was on this combination for around six months, additionally suffering from insomnia, often not being able to sleep until 4 am and then rising again at 7 am. Within two months of taking her CBD oil, as well as a topical CBD salve, she was able to sleep through the night, from around 10.30 pm until almost 6 am, uninterrupted. She also used to find that she woke up during the night with bladder control issues and needing to pee; however, this also improved after commencing her CBD regime. This patient additionally reported suffering with fibromyalgia and migraines, as well as anxiety. All conditions were managed solely with the CBD sublingual products and topical balm with the odd addition of ibuprofen if the pain got unbearable.

BIBLIOGRAPHY

Aldrich, M. (1997). History of therapeutic cannabis. In: M. L. Mathre (Ed.), *Cannabis in Medical Practice: A Legal, Historical and Pharmacological Overview of the Therapeutic Use of Marijuana* (pp. 35–55). London: McFarland.

Alzoubi, K. H., Al Hilo, A. S., Al-Balas, Q. A., El-Salem, K., El-Elimat, T., & Alali, F. Q. (2019). Withania somnifera root powder protects against post-traumatic stress disorder-induced memory impairment. *Molecular Biology Reports*, June: 4709–4715.

Amada, N., Yamasaki, Y., Williams, C. M., & Whalley, B. J. (2013). Cannabidivarin (CBDV) suppresses pentylenetetrazole (PTZ)-induced increases in epilepsy-related gene expression. *PeerJ*, 21 November. 20 September 2020. What is the second date?

Andrew, C. M., Hausman, J.-F., & Guerriero, G. (2016). Cannabis sativa: the plant of the thousand and one molecules. *Frontiers in Plant Science*: 7–19.

Appendino, G., Gibbons, S., Giana, A., Pagani, A., Grassi, G., Stavri, M., Smith, E., & Mukhlesur Rahman, M. (2008). Antibacterial cannabinoids from Cannabis sativa: a structure-activity study. *Journal of Natural Products*: 1427–1430.

Arseneault, L., Cannon, M., Witton, J., & Murray, R. M. (2004). Causal association between cannabis and psychosis: examination of the evidence. *British Journal of Psychiatry*, 184(2): 110–117.

Auddy, B., Hazra, J., & Nagar, B. (2008). A standardized Withania somnifera extract significantly reduces stress-related parameters in chronically stressed humans: a double-blind, randomized, placebo-controlled study. *Journal of the American Nutraceutical Association*: 50–56.

Bahi, A., Al Mansouri, S., Al Memari, E., Al Ameri, M., Nurulain, S. M., & Ojha, S. (2014). β-Caryophyllene, a CB-2 receptor agonist produces multiple behavioral changes relevant to anxiety and depression in mice. *Physiology & Behaviour*, August: 119–124.

Batra, P., & Sharma, A. K. (2013). Anti-cancer potential of flavonoids: recent trends and future perspectives. *3 Biotech*, December: 439–459.

Benito, C., Nunez, E., Tolon, R. M., Carrier, E. J., Rabano, A., Hillard, C. J., & Romero, J. (2003). Cannabinoid CB-2 receptors and fatty acid amide hydrolase are selectively overexpressed in neuritic plaque-associated glia in Alzheimer's disease brains. *Journal of Neuroscience*: 11136–11141.

Bento da Silva, M. T., Brandim Marques, R., Batista-Lima, F. J., Almeida Soares, M., Aguiaar dos Santos, A., Caldas Magalhaes, P. J., de Assis Oliveira, F., & de Castro Almeida, F. R. (2016). α-terpineol induces gastric retention of liquids by inhibiting vagal parasympathetic pathways in rats. *Planta Medica*, October: 1329–1334.

Bian, G., Ma, T., & Liu, T. (2018). In vivo platforms for terpenoid overproduction and the generation of chemical diversity. *Methods in Enzymology*, 608: 97–129.

Bluett, R. J., Gamble-George, J. C., Hermanson, D. J., Hartley, N. D., Marnett, L. J., & Patel, S. (2014). Central anandamide deficiency predicts stress-induced anxiety: behavioral reversal through endocannabinoid augmentation. *Translational Psychiatry*, 4: e408.

Bolognini, D., Costa, B., Maione, S., Comelli, F., Marini, P., Di Marzo, V., Parolaro, D., Ross, R. A., Gauson, L. A., Cascio, M. G., & Pertwee, R. G. (2010). The plant cannabinoid Delta9-tetrahydrocannabivarin can decrease signs of inflammation and inflammatory pain in mice. *British Journal of Pharmacology*: 677–687.

Bonamina, F., Moraes, T. M., dos Santosa, R. C., Kushima, H., Faria, F. M., Silva, M. A., Junior, I. V., Nogueira, L., Bauab, T. M., Alba, R. M., Brito, S., da Rocha, L. R. M., & Hiruma-Lima, C. A. (2014). The effect of a minor constituent of essential oil from

Citrus aurantium: the role of β-myrcene in preventing peptic ulcer disease. *Chemico-Biological Interactions*: 11–19.

Borgelt, L. M., Franson, K. L., Nussbaum, A. M., & Wang, G. S. (2013). The pharmacologic and clinical effects of medical cannabis. *Pharmacotherapy*: 195–209.

Borrelli, F., Pagano, E., Romano, B., Panzera, S., Maiello, F., Coppola, D., De Petrocellis, L., Buono, L., Orlando, P., & Izzo, A. A. (2013). Colon carcinogenesis is inhibited by the TRPM8 antagonist cannabigerol, a Cannabis-derived non-psychotropic cannabinoid. *Carcinogenesis*: 2787–2797.

Brill, H., & Nahas, G. G. (1984). Cannabis intoxication and mental illness. In: Nahas, G. G., *Marijuana in Science and Medicine* (pp. 263–306). New York: Raven.

Broyd, N. (2020). Long COVID defined ahead of UK guidelines. *Medscape*, 30 October. 02 November 2020. Second date?

Carlini, E. A., Karniol, I. G., Renault, P. F., & Schuster, C. R. (1974). Effects of Marihuana in laboratory animals and in man. *British Journal of Pharmacology*, 50(2): 299–309.

Carrillo-Salinas, F. J., Navarrete, C., Mecha, M., Feliú, A., Collado, J. A., Cantarero, I., Bellido, M. L., Muñoz, E., & Guaza, C. (2014). A cannabigerol derivative suppresses immune responses and protects mice from experimental autoimmune encephalomyelitis. *PLoS One*, 9(4): e94733.

Casano, S., Grassi, G., Martini, V., & Michelozzi, M. (2011). Variations in terpene profiles of different strains of Cannabis sativa L. *International Society for Horticultural Science*, 10 April. Second date?

Chaves, J. C., Leal, P. C., Pianowisky, L., & Calixto, J. B. (2008). Pharmacokinetics and tissue distribution of the sesquiterpene alpha-humulene in mice. *Planta Medica*, October: 1678–1683.

Chen, H., Yuan, J., Hao, J., Wen, Y., Lv, Y., Chen, L., & Yang, X. (2019). α-humulene inhibits hepatocellular carcinoma cell proliferation and induces apoptosis through the inhibition of Akt signaling. *Food and Chemical Toxicology*, September.

Cheng, W.-W., Lin, C.-T., Chu, F.-H., Chang, S.-T., & Wang, S.-Y. (2009). Neuropharmacological activities of phytoncide released from Cryptomeria japonica. *Journal of Wood Science*, February: 27–31.

Cogan, P. S. (2020). The "entourage effect" or "hodge-podge hashish": the questionable rebranding, marketing, and expectations of cannabis polypharmacy. *Expert Review of Clinical Pharmacology*: 835–845.

DeLong, G. T., Wolf, C. E., Poklis, A., & Lichtman, A. H. (2010). Pharmacological evaluation of the natural constituent of Cannabis sativa, cannabichromene and its modulation by Δ(9)-tetrahydrocannabinol. *Drug and Alcohol Dependence*: 126–133.

de Moraisa, H., de Souzaa, C. P., da Silva, L. M., Ferreira, D. M., Hatsuko Baggio, C., Vanvossen, A. C., de Carvalhoc, M. C., Silva-Santos, J. E., Bertoglio, L. J., Cunhaa, J. M., & Zanovelia, J. M. (2016). Anandamide reverses depressive-like behavior, neurochemical abnormalities and oxidative-stress parameters in streptozotocin-diabetic rats: Role of CB-1 receptors. *European Neuropsychopharmacology*: 1590–1600.

Dietrich, A., & McDaniel, W. F. (2004). Endocannabinoids and exercise. *British Journal of Sports Medicine*: 536–541.

Duncombe, S. (2017). Indica vs. sativa: what's the difference? *Leaf Science*, 16 October. 10 August 2019.

Duncombe, S. (2017). What are the medical benefits of CBD? *Leaf Science*, 6 December. 10 June 2020.

Duncombe, S. (2018). What is clinical endocannabinoid deficiency? *Leaf Science*, 25 January. 10 June 2020. Why two dates in each of the three above listings (all relocated to author)?

DuToit, B. M. (1980). *Cannabis in Africa: A Survey of Its Distribution in Africa and a Study of Cannabis Use and Users in Multi-ethnic South Africa*. Rotterdam, the Netherlands: A. A. Bolkema.

El-Alfy, A. T., Ivey, K., Robinson, K., Ahmed, S., Radwan, M., Slade, D., Khan, I., ElSohly, M., & Ross, S. (2010). Antidepressant-like effect of delta9-tetrahydrocannabinol and other cannabinoids isolated from Cannabis sativa L. *Pharmacology, Biochemistry, and Behavior*: 434–442.

Elzinga,S., Fischedick, J., Podkolonski, R., & Raber, J. C. (2015). Cannabinoids and terpenes as chemotaxonomic markers in Cannabis. *Natural Products Chemistry and Research*, 3(4): 1–9.

Erukainure, O. L., Kayode, F. O., Adeyoju, O. A., Adenekan, S. O., Asieba, G., Ajayi, A., Adegbola, M. V., & Sarumi, B. B. (2015). Antioxidant and chemical properties of essential oil extracted from blend of selected spices. *Journal of Coastal Life Medicine*: 575–578.

Esposito, G., Pesce, M., Seguella, L., Sanseverino, W., Lu, J., Corpetti, C., & Sarnelli, G. (2020). The potential of cannabidiol in the COVID-19 pandemic. *British Journal of Pharmacology*, July: 4967–4970.

Eubanks, L. M., Rogers, C. J., Beuscher, A. E. 4th, Koob, G. F., Olson, A. J., Dickerson, T. J., & Janda, K. D. (2006). A molecular link between the active component of marijuana and Alzheimer's disease pathology. *Molecular Pharmaceutics*, 3(6): 773–777.

Falk, A., Lof, A., Hagberg, M., Wigaeus Hjelm, E., & Wang, Z. (1991). Human exposure to 3-carene by inhalation: toxicokinetics, effects on pulmonary function and occurrence of irritative and CNS symptoms. *Toxicology and Applied Pharmacology*: 198–205.

Fankhauser, M. (2002). History of Cannabis in Western medicine. In: E. B. Russo & F. Grotenhermen (Eds.),. *Cannabis and Cannabinoids: Pharmacology, Toxicology and Therapeutic Potential* (pp. 37–38). New York: Haworth.

Fine, P. G., & Rosenfeld, M. J. (2013). The endocannabinoid system, cannabinoids, and pain. *Rambam Maimonides Medical Journal*, October: e0022.

Fisher, E., Eccleston, C., Degenhardt, L., Finn, D. P., Finnerup, N. B., Gilron, I., Haroutounian, S., Krane, E., Rice, A. S. C., Rowbotham, M., Wallace, M., & Moore, A. R. (2019). Cannabinoids, cannabis, and cannabis-based medicine for pain management: a protocol for an overview of systematic reviews and a systematic review of randomised controlled trials. *Pain Reports*: e741.

Fuss, J., Steinle, J., Bindila, L., Auer, M. K., Kirchherr, H., Lutz, B., & Gass, P. (2015). A runner's high depends on cannabinoid receptors in mice. *Proceedings of the National Academy of Sciences of the United States of America (PNAS)*, 112(42): 13105–13108.

Gamble, L. J., Boesch, J. M., Frye, C. W., Schwark, W. S., Mann, S., Wolfe, L., Brown, H., Berthelsen, E. S., & Wakschlag, J. J. (2018). Pharmacokinetics, safety, and clinical efficacy of cannabidiol treatment in osteoarthritic dogs. *Frontiers in Veterinary Science*, July.

Gaoni, Y., & Mechoulam, R. (1964). Isolation, structure and partial synthesis of an active constituent of hashish. *Journal of the American Chemical Society, 86*: 1646–1647.

García, C., Palomo-Garo, C., García-Arencibia, M., Ramos, J. A., Pertwee, R. G., & Fernández-Ruiz, J. (2011). Symptom-relieving and neuroprotective effects of the phytocannabinoid Δ^9-THCV in animal models of Parkinson's disease. *British Journal of Pharmacology*: 1495–1506.

Gertsch, J., Leonti, M., Raduner, S., Racz, I., Chen, J.-Z., Xie, X.-Q., Altmann, K.-H., Karsak, M., & Zimmer, A. (2008). Beta-caryophyllene is a dietary cannabinoid. *Proceedings of the National Academy of Sciences of the United States of America (PNAS)*, July.

Green, K. (1998). Marijuana smoking vs cannabinoids for glaucoma therapy. *Archives of Opthalmology, 11*: 1433–1477.

Greenwell, G. T. (2012). Medical marijuana use for chronic pain: risks and benefits. *Journal of Pain and Palliative Care Pharmacotherapy, 26*(1): 68–69.

Grinspoon, L. (1971). *Marijuana Reconsidered*. Cambridge, MA: Harvard University Press.

Grinspoon, L., & Bakalar, J. B. (1993). *Marijuana the Forbidden Medicine*. New Haven, CT: Yale University Press.

Grotenhermen, F., Leson, G., & Pless, P. (2003). Evaluating the impact of THC in hemp foods and cosmetics on human health & workplace drug tests. *Journal of Industrial Hemp, 8*: 5–36.

Gupta, M., & Kaur, G. (2019). Withania somnifera (L.) Dunal ameliorates neurodegeneration and cognitive impairments associated with systemic inflammation. *BMC Complementary and Alternative Medicine*, August: Article No. 217.

Hampson, A. J., Axelrod, J., & Grimaldi, M. (1999). Cannabinoids as antioxidants and neuroprotectants. United States: Patent US6630507B1. Publisher?

Hassannia, B., Logie, E., Vandenabeele, P., Vanden Berghe, T., & Vanden Berghe, W. (2020). Withaferin A: from ayurvedic folk medicine to preclinical anti-cancer drug. *Biochemical Pharmacology*, March: 113602.

Hau, D. C., & Xiao, P. G. (2015). Phytochemical and biological research of Cannabis pharmaceutical resources. *Medicinal Plants—Chemistry, Biology and Omics*: 431–464.

Heyman, E., Gamelin, F. X., Goekint, M., Piscitelli, F., Roelands, B., Leclair, E., Di Marzo, V., & Meeusen, R. (2012). Intense exercise increases circulating endocannabinoid and BDNF levels in humans—possible implications for reward and depression. *Psychoneuroendocrinology*: 844–851.

Horváth, B., Mukhopadhyay, P., Kechrid, M., Patel, V., Tanashian, G., Wink, D. A., Gertsch, J., & Pacher, P. (2012). β-caryophyllene ameliorates cisplatin-induced nephrotoxicity in a cannabinoid 2 receptor-dependent manner. *Free Radical Biology and Medicine*, April: 1325–1333.

Hsu, C.-C., Lai, W.-L., Chuang, K.-C., Lee, M.-H., & Tsai, Y.-C. (2013). The inhibitory activity of linalool against the filamentous growth and biofilm formation in Candida albicans. *Medical Mycology*: 473–482.

Izzo, A. A. (2004). Cannabinoids and intestinal motility: welcome to CB-2 receptors. *British Journal of Pharmacology*: 1201–1202.

Jeena, K., Liju, V. B., Umadevi, N. P., & Kuttan, R. (2014). Antioxidant, anti-inflammatory and antinociceptive properties of black pepper essential oil (Piper nigrum Linn.). *Journal of Essential Oil Bearing Plants*: 1–12.

Jeong, J.-G., Kim, Y. S., Min, Y. K., & Kim, S. H. (2008). Low concentration of 3-carene stimulates the differentiation of mouse osteoblastic MC3T3-E1 subclone 4 cells. *Phytotherapy Research*, January: 18–22.

Jones, N. A., Hill, A. J., Smith, I., Bevan, S. A., WIlliams, C. M., Whalley, B. J., & Stephens, G. J. (2010). Cannabidiol displays antiepileptiform and antiseizure properties in vitro and in vivo. *Journal of Pharmacology and Experimental Therapeutics*, 332(2): 569–577.

Kandel, D. B. (1984). Marijuana users in young adulthood. *Archives of General Psychiatry*: 200–209.

Kasiri, N., Rahmati, M., Ahmadi, L., & Eskandari, N. (2018). The significant impact of apigenin on different aspects of autoimmune disease. *Inflammopharmacology*, December: 1359–1373.

Kerba, M. (2019). Strong reasons make strong actions: medical cannabis and cancer—a call for collective action. *Current Oncology*, June: 160–161.

Kleckner, A. S., Kleckner, I. R., Kamen, C. S., Tejani, M. A., Janelsins, M. C., Morrow, G. R., & Peppone, L. J. (2019).

Opportunities for cannabis in supportive care in cancer. *Therapeutic Advances in Medical Oncology*, August.

Komorowski, J., & Stepien, H. (2007). The role of the endocannabinoid system in the regulation of endocrine function and in the control of energy balance in humans. *Postepy Higieny i medycyny doswiadczalnej*: 99–105.

Konieczny, E., & Wilson, L. (2018). *Healing with CBD*. Berkeley, CA: Ulysses.

Kruk-Slomka, M., Michalak, A., & Biala, G. (2015). Antidepressant-like effects of the cannabinoid receptor ligands in the forced swimming test in mice: mechanism of action and possible interactions with cholinergic system. *Behavioural Brain Research*: 24–36.

LaLone, C. A., Hammer, K. D. P., Wu, L., Bae, J., Leyva, N., Liu, Y., Solco, A. K. S., Kraus, G. A., Murphy, P. A., Wurtele, E. S., Kim, O.-K., Widrlechner, M. P., & Birt, D. F. (2007). Echinacea species and alkamides inhibit prostaglandin E2 production in RAW264.7 mouse macrophage cells. *Journal of Agricultural Food and Chemistry*, August: 7314–7322.

Li, H.-L. (1973). An archeological and historical account of cannabis in China. *Economic Botany*, 28: 437–448.

Li, H. L. (1978). Hallucinogenic plants in Chinese herbals. *Journal of Psychedelic Drugs*, 10(1): 17–26.

Lipari, R. N., Hedden, S. L., & Hughes, A. (2014). *Substance Use and Mental Health Estimates from the 2013 National Survey on Drug Use and Health—Overview of Findings*. US Dept of Health & Human Services Report. Rockville, MD: Center for Behavioral Health Statistics and Quality (CBHSQ).

Lisboa, S. F., Borges, A. A., Nejo, P., Fassini, A., Guimaraes, F. S., & Resstel, L. B. (2015). Cannabinoid CB-1 receptors in the dorsal hippocampus and prelimbic medial prefrontal cortex modulate anxiety-like behavior in rats: additional evidence. *Progress in Neuro-psychopharmacology & Biological Psychiatry*: 76–83.

Lopes Salles, E., Khodadadi, H., Jarrahi, A., Ahluwalia, M., Paffaro, V. A., Costigliola, V., Yu, J. C., Hess, D. C., Dhandapani, K. M., & Baban, B. (2020). Cannabidiol (CBD) modulation of apelin in acute respiratory distress syndrome. *Journal of Cellular and Molecular Medicine*, October.

Lopresti, A. L., Drummond, P. D., & Smith, S. J. (2019). A randomized, double-blind, placebo-controlled, crossover study examining the hormonal and vitality effects of ashwagandha (Withania somnifera) in aging, overweight males. *American Journal of Men's Health*, March–April.

Ludwiczuk, A., & Georgiev, M. I. (2017). Terpenoids. *Pharmacognosy—Fundamentals, Applications and Strategies*: 233–266.

Ma, J., Xu, H., Wu, J., Qu, C., Sun, F., & Xu, S. (2015). Linalool inhibits cigarette smoke-induced lung inflammation by inhibiting NF-κB activation. *International Immunopharmacology*: 708–713.

Maccarrone, M., Lorenzon, T., Bari, M., Melino, G., & Finazzi-Agrò, A. (2000). Anandamide induces apoptosis in human cells via vanilloid receptors—evidence for a protective role of cannabinoid receptors. *Journal of Biological Chemistry*: 1741–1750.

Malavazi de Christo Scherer, M., Martins Marques, F., Moreira Figueira, M., Oliveira Peisino, M. C., Pimentel Schmitt, E. F., Kondratyuk, T., Countinho Endringer, D., Scherer, R., & Fronza, M. (2019). Wound healing activity of terpinolene and α-phellandrene by attenuating inflammation and oxidative stress in vitro. *Journal of Tissue Viability*, May: 94–99.

Maoine, S., Piscitelli, F., Gatta, L., Vita, D., De Petrocellis, L., Palazzo, E., de Novellis, V., & Di Marzo, V. (2011). Non-psychoactive cannabinoids modulate the descending pathway of antinociception in anaesthetized rats through several mechanisms of action. *British Journal Pharmacology*: 584–596.

Martin, B. R., Mechoulam, R., & Razdam, R. K. (1999). Discovery and characterization of endogenous cannabinoids. *Life Sciences*, 65(6–7): 573–595.

McPartland, J., & Russo, E. B. (2001). Cannabis and Cannabis extracts: greater than the sum of their parts? Researchgate.net, June. 11 April 2018. Why second date?

Mechoulam, R. (1973). *Marijuana: Chemistry, Pharmacology, Metabolism and Clinical Effects*. New York: Academic Press.

Mechoulam, R., Berry, E. M., Avraham, Y., DiMarzo, V., & Fride, E. (2006). Endocannabinoids, feeding and suckling—from our perspective. *International Journal of Obesity*, Suppl. 1: S24–S28.

MedicalJane (n.d.). Terpenes—learn how terpenes work synergisticaslly with cannabinoids. https://medicaljane.com/category/cannabis-classroom/terpenes/. 3 April 2018.

Mielnik, C. A., Lam, V. M., & Ross, R. A. (2020). CB-1 allosteric modulators and their therapeutic potential in CNS disorders. *Progress in Neuro-Psychopharmacology and Biological Psychiatry*, November.

Mikuriya, T. H. (1969). Marijuana in medicine: past, present and future. *California Medicine*, 110(1): 34–40.

Musto, D. F. (1972). The Marijuana Tax Act of 1937. *Archive of General Psychiatry*: 101–108.

Nabavi, S. F., Braidy, N., Gortzi, O., Sobarzo-Sanchez, E., Daglia, M., Skalicka-Wozniak, K., & Nabavi, S. M. (2015). Luteolin as an anti-inflammatory and neuroprotective agent: a brief review. *Brain Research Bulletin*, October: 1–11.

Nahas, G. G., & Paris, M. (1984). Botany: the unstabilized species. In: G. G. Nahas (Ed.), *Marijuana in Science and Medicine* (pp. 3–36). New York: Raven.

National Toxicology Program Technical Report Series. (1996). *NTP Toxicology and Carcinogenesis Studies of 1-Trans-Delta(9)-Tetrahydrocannabinol (CAS No. 1972-08-3) in F344 Rats and B6C3F1 Mice (Gavage Studies)*. Publisher?

Nehlig, A. (2013). The neuroprotective effects of cocoa flavanol and its influence on cognitive performance. *British Journal of Clinical Pharmacology*: 716–727.

Okumura, N., Yoshida, H., Nishimura, Y., Kitagishi, Y., & Matsuda, S. (2011). Terpinolene, a component of herbal sage, downregulates AKT1 expression in K562 cells. *Oncology Letters*: 321–324.

Ortiz de Urbina, A. V., Martin, M. L., Montero, M. J., Moran, A., & San Roman, L. (1989). Sedating and antipyretic activity of the essential oil of Calamintha sylvatica subsp. ascendens. *Journal of Ethnopharmacology*: 165–171.

Pacher, P., & Mechoulam, R. (2011). Is lipid signaling through cannabinoid 2 receptors part of a protective system? *Progress in Lipid Research*: 193–211.

Parker, L. A., Rock, E. M., & Limebeer, C. L. (2011). Regulation of nausea and vomiting by cannabinoids. *British Journal of Pharmacology*, 163(7): 1411–1422.

Patel, S., & Hillard, C. J. (2009). Role of endocannabinoid signaling in anxiety and depression. *Current Topics in Behavioural Neurosciences*: 347–371.

Patsos, H. A., Hicks, D. J., Dobson, R. R. H., Greenhough, A., Woodman, N., Lane, J. D., Williams, A. C., & Paraskeva, C. (2005). The endogenous cannabinoid, anandamide, induces cell death in colorectal carcinoma cells: a possible role for cyclooxygenase 2. *Gut*: 1741–1750.

PDQ Cancer Complementary and Alternative Medicine Editorial Board. (2016). NCBI Bookshelf. A service of the National Library of Medicine, National Institutes of Health. 8 January 2016. 8 June 2020. Double dating! https://ncbi.nlm.nih.gov/books/NBK65875.3/?report=printable. Add date last accessed—8 June 2020?

Persidsky, Y., Fan, S., Dykstra, H., Reichenbach, N. L., Rom, S., & Ramirez, S. H. (2015). 1. Persidsky Y. activation of cannabinoid type two receptors diminish inflammatory responses in macrophages and brain endothelium. *Journal of Neuroimmune Pharmacology*: 302–308.

Pertwee, R. G. (2001). Cannabinoid Receptors and Pain." *Progress in Neurobiology*, 63(5): 569–611.

de Pinho, A. R. (2016). Social and medical aspects of the use of Cannabis in Brazil. *Semantic Scholar*, 7 June 2020. Second date—meaning?

Pope, H. G. Jr, Gruber, A. J., Hudson, J. I., Cohane, G., Huestis, M. A., & Yurgelun-Todd, D. (2003). Early-onset cannabis use and cognitive deficits: what is the nature of the association? *Drug and Alcohol Dependence*, 69(3): 303–310.

Prasad, B., Radulovacki, M. G., & Carley, D. W. (2013). Proof of concept trial of dronabinol in obstructive sleep apnea. *Frontiers in Psychiatry*, 4(1).

Rapino, C., Battista, N., Bari, M., & Macarronne, M. (2014). Endocannabinoids as biomarkers of human reproduction. *Human Reproduction Update*: 501–516.

Rock, E. M., Sticht, M. A., Duncan, M., Stott, C., & Parker, L. A. (2013). Evaluation of the potential of the phytocannabinoids, cannabidivarin (CBDV) and Δ9-tetrahydrocannabivarin (THCV), to produce CB-1 receptor inverse agonism symptoms of nausea in rats. *British Journal of Pharmacology*: 671–678.

Rogerio, A. P., Andrade, E. L., Leite, D. F. P., Figueiredo, C. P., & Calixto, J. B. (2009). Preventive and therapeutic anti-inflammatory properties of the sesquiterpene alpha-humulene in experimental airways allergic inflammation. *British Journal of Pharmacology*, October: 1074–1087.

Rohr, A. C., Wilkins, C. K., Clausen, P. A., Hammer, M., Nielsen, G. D., Wolkoff, P., & Spengler, J. D. (2002). Upper airway and pulmonary effects of oxidation products of (+)- α-pinene, d-limonene, and isoprene in balm/C mice. *Inhalation Toxicology*, 14(7).

Romano, B., Borrelli, F., Fasolino, I., Capasso, R., Piscitelli, F., Cascio, M., Pertwee, R., Coppola, D., Vassalo, L., Orlando, P., Di Marzo, V., & Izzo, A. (2013). The cannabinoid TRPA1 agonist cannabichromene inhibits nitric oxide production in macrophages and ameliorates murine colitis. *British Journal of Pharmacology*: 213–229.

Rufino, A. T., Ribeiro, M., Judas, F., Salguerio, L., Lopes, M. C., Cavaleiro, C., & Mendes, A. F. (2014). Anti-inflammatory and chondroprotective activity of (+)- α-pinene: structural and enantiomeric selectivity. *Journal of Natural Products*, January: 264–269.

Russo, E. B. (2011). Taming THC: potential cannabis synergy and phytocannabinoid-terpenoid entourage effects. *British Journal of Pharmacology*: 1344–1364.

Russo, E. B., & Guy, G. W. (2005). A tale of two cannabinoids: the therapeutic rationale for combining tetrahydrocannabinol and cannabidiol. *Medical Hypotheses*: 234–246.

Russo, E. B., & Marcu, J. (2017). Cannabis pharmacology: the usual suspects and a few promising leads. *Advanced Pharmacology*, June: 67–134.

Sabogal-Guaqueta, A. M., Osorio, E., & Cardona-Gomez, G. P. (2016). Linalool reverses neuropathological and behavioral impairments in old triple transgenic Alzheimer's mice. *Neuropharmacology*, March: 111–120.

Salehi, B., Venditti, A., Sharifi-Rad, M., Kregiel, D., Sharifi-Rad, J., Durazzo, A., Lucarini, M., Santini, A., Souto, E. B., Novellino, E., Antolak, H., Azzini, E., Setzer, W. N., & Martins, N. (2019). The therapeutic potential of apigenin. *International Journal of Molecular Sciences*, March: 1305.

Sawler, J., Stout, J. M., Gardner, K. M., Hudson, D., Vidmar, J., Butler, L., Page, J. E., & Myles, S. (2015). The genetic structure of marijuana and hemp. *PLoS One*.

Schiller, H., Forster, A., Vonhoff, C., Hegger, M., Biller, A., & Winterhoff, H. (2006). Sedating effects of Humulus lupulus L. extracts. *Phytomedicine*, September: 535–541.

Shinjyo, N., & Di Marzo, V. (2013). The effect of cannabichromene on adult neural stem/progenitor cells. *Neurochemistry International*: 432–437.

Siqueira, H. D'A. S., Neto, B. S., Sousa, D. P., Gomes, B. S., da Silva, F. V., Cunha, F. V. M., Wanderley, C. W. S., Pinheiro, G., Candido, A., Wong, D., Ribeiro, R., Lima-Junior, R., & Oliveira, F. (2016). α-phellandrene, a cyclic monoterpene, attenuates inflammatory response through neutrophil migration inhibition and mast cell degranulation. *Life Sciences*: 27–33.

Steep Hill Laboratories (2014). https://steephill.com/science/terpenes (last accessed 10 April 2018). Is this right?

Touw, M. (1981). The religious and medicinal uses of Cannabis in China, India and Tibet. *Journal of Psychoactive Drugs*, 13(1): 23–34.

Turner, C. E., & Elsohly, M. A. (1981). Biological activity of cannabichromene, its homologs and isomers. *Journal of Clinical Pharmacology*.

Valdeolivas, S., Navarrete, C., Cantarero, I., Bellido, M. L., Munoz, E., & Sagredo, O. (2015). Neuroprotective properties of cannabigerol in Huntington's disease: studies in R6/2 mice and 3-nitropropionate-lesioned mice. *Neurotherapeutics*: 185–199.

Valente, J., Zuzarte, M., Liberal, J., Goncalves, M. J., Lopes, M. C., Cavaleiro, C., Cruz, M. T., & Salgueiro, L. (2013). Margotia gummifera essential oil as a source of anti-inflammatory drugs. *Industrial Crops and Products*: 86–91.

Vallianou, I., Peroulis, N., Pantazis, P., & Hadzopoulou-Cladaras, M. (2011). Camphene, a plant-derived monoterpene, reduces plasma cholesterol and triglycerides in hyperlipidemic rats independently of HMG-CoA reductase activity. *PLoS Ome*: e20516.

Varga, Z. V., Matyas, C., Erdelyi, K., Cinar, R., Nieri, D., Chicca, A., Nemeth, B. T., Paloczi, J., Lajtos, T., Corey, L., Hasko, G., Gao, B., Kunos, G., Gertsch, J., & Pachercorrespo, P. (2018). β-caryophyllene protects against alcoholic steatohepatitis by attenuating inflammation and metabolic dysregulation in mice. *British Journal of Pharmacology*, January: 320–334.

Visavadiya, N. P., & Narasimhacharya, A. V. R. L. (2007). Hypocholesteremic and antioxidant effects of Withania somnifera (Dunal) in hypercholesteremic rats. *Phytomedicine*, February: 136–142.

Walker, J. M., Huang, S. M., Strangman, N. M., Tsou, K., & Sañudo-Peña, M. C. (1999). Pain modulation by release of the endogenous cannabinoid anandamide. *Proceedings of the National Academy of Sciences of the United States of America*, 96(21): 12198–12203.

Wargent, E. T., Zaibi, M. S., Silvestri, C., Hislop, D., C. Stocker, C, J., Stott, C. G., Guy, G. W., Duncan, M., Di Marzo, V., & Cawthorne, M. A. (2013). The cannabinoid Δ(9)-tetrahydrocannabivarin (THCV) ameliorates insulin sensitivity in two mouse models of obesity. *Nutrition & Diabetes*: e68.

Wasserman, E., Tam, J., Mechoulam, R., Zimmer, A., Maor, G., & Bab, I. (2015). CB-1 cannabinoid receptors mediate endochondral skeletal growth attenuation by Δ9-tetrahydrocannabinol. *Annals of the New York Academy of Sciences*.

Weiqiang, C., Ying, L., Ming, L., Jianwen, M., Lirong, Z., Rongbo, H., Xiaobao, J., & Lianbao, Y. (2015). Anti-tumor effect of α-pinene on human hepatoma cell lines through inducing G2/M cell cycle arrest. *Journal of Pharmacological Sciences*, March: 332–338.

Wiley Online Library (2005, 14 June). Conversation with Elisaldo Luiz de Araújo Carlini (E. A. Carlini). 7 June 2020. Date last accessed? Add URL.

Wilkinson, J. D., Whalley, B. J., Baker, D., Pryce, G., Contantini, A., Gibbons, S., & Williamson, E. M. (2003). Medicinal cannabis:

is delta9-tetrahydrocannabinol necessary for all its effects? *Journal of Pharmacy and Pharmacology*: 1687–1694.

Woelkart, K., Xu, W., Pei, Y., Makriyannis, A., Picone, R. P., & Bauer, R. (2005). The endocannabinoid system as a target for alkamides from Echinacea angustifolia roots. *Planta Medica*, August: 701–705.

Wolfe, D., & Holdstock, S. (2005). *Naked Chocolate—The Astonishing Truth about the World's Greatest Food*. Berkeley, CA: North Atlantic.

Yamaori, S., Ebisawa, J., Okushima, Y., Yamamoto, I., & Watanabe, K. (2011). Potent inhibition of human cytochrome P450 3A isoforms by cannabidiol: role of phenolic hydroxyl groups in the resorcinol moiety. *Life Sciences*: 730–736.

Yang, I., Li, F.-F., Han, Y.-C., Jia, B., & Ding, Y. (2015). Cannabinoid receptor CB-2 is involved in tetrahydrocannabinol-induced anti-inflammation against lipopolysaccharide in MG-63 cells. *Mediators of Inflammation*.

Yoshida, H., Usami, N., Ohishi, Y., Watenabe, K., Yamamoto, I., & Yoshimura, H. (1995). Synthesis and pharmacological effects in mice of halogenated cannabinol derivatives. *Chemical & Pharmaceutical Bulletin (Tokyo)*: 335–337.

Zanelati, T. V., Biojone, C., Moreira, F. A., Guimaraes, F. S., & Joca, S. R. L. (2010). Antidepressant-like effects of cannabidiol in mice: possible involvement of 5-HT1A receptors. *British Journal of Pharmacology*, 159(1): 122–128.

Zendulka, O., Dovrtělová, G., Nosková, K., Turjap, M., Šulcová, A., Hanuš, L., & Juřica, J. (2016). Cannabinoids and cytochrome P450 interactions. *Current Drug Metabolism*: 206–226.

Zhang, X., Qin, Y., Pan, Z., Li, M., Liu, X., Chen, X., Qu, G., Zhou, L., Xu, M., Zheng, Q., & Li, D. (2019). Cannabidiol induces cell cycle arrest and cell apoptosis in human gastric cancer SGC-7901 cells. *Biomolecules*, July: 302.

Zuardi, A. W. (2006). History of cannabis as medicine: a review. *Brazilian Journal of Psychiatry*, 28(2): 153–157.

INDEX

Actea racemosa. See black cohosh
ADD. *See* attention deficit disorder
ADHD. *See* attention deficit hyperactivity disorder
adult respiratory distress syndrome (ARDS), 155
AEA. *See* N-arachidonoy-lethanolamine
2-AG. *See* 2-arachidonylgylycerol
alkamides, 96
alveoli, 139
amenorrhoea, 142
amygdale, 39
anandamide, 11, 22, 36
   breast milk, 26
   cell regulation and development, 26
   effects upon body, 23
   increasing level in body, 27
   mood enhancement, 25
   pain relief, 24
   pleasure hormone, 24
   reproduction and fertility, 25
   retrograde transmission, 23–24
   role of, 24
   runner's high, 24–25

anthocyanidins, 86. *See also* flavonoids
anthoxanthins, 85. *See also* flavonoids
antibiotics, 122–123. *See also* canabidiol contraindications
antidepressants and anti-anxiety medicines, 123. *See also* canabidiol contraindications
antinociceptive, 75
antioxidant mushrooms, 99
anxiety, 130–133. *See also* health conditions and CBD
   anti-anxiety medicines, 123
   and post cancer malaise, 164–165
apelin, 156
apigenin, 90. *See also* flavonoids
apoptosis. *See* cell death
2-arachidonylgylycerol (2-AG), 36
ARDS. *See* adult respiratory distress syndrome
aromadendrin, 87. *See also* flavonoids

arthritis, 133. *See also* health conditions and CBD
aryophyllene, 73–75. *See also* plant secondary metabolites
ashwagandha (*Withania somnifera*), 97. *See also* herbal synergy
   cannabis and, 97–98
   synergy between CBD and, 98–99
attention deficit disorder (ADD), 129–130
attention deficit hyperactivity disorder (ADHD), 129–130
auto phagocytosis, 91
Avicenna. *See* Ibn Sina

BCP. *See* beta-caryophyllene
Behçet's disease, 135–136. *See also* health conditions and CBD
Behçet's syndrome. *See* Behçet's disease
beta-caryophyllene (BCP), 94
black cohosh (*Cimicifuga racemosa* or *Actea racemosa*), 96. *See also* herbal synergy
blood thinners, 123. *See also* canabidiol contraindications
bronchioles, 138
butin, 87. *See also* flavonoids

cacao, 100–101. *See also* herbal synergy
cake analogy, 17, 65
camphene, 79–80. *See also* plant secondary metabolites
canabidiol (CBD), xiii, 1, 20, 53, 92. *See also Cannabis sativa*
   anandamide, 11
   as anti-inflammatory agent, 154
   cannabis resin, 6
   effects in pets, 105–108
   endocannabinoid system deficiency, 11
   interaction with endocannabinoid system, 42–43
   medicinal properties 21–22
   modern thinking, 10–12
   nineteenth and twentieth centuries, 5–9
   oil, 12
   post-Christianity, 4–5
   products, xv
   purchasing, 109–113
   synergy between ashwagandha and, 98–99
   prior to Christianity, 2–4
   UK marketplace, 109
   uses of hemp, 1
   in western medical use, 9–10
canabidiol benefits, 13
   anxiety, 14
   general well-being, 14
   joint pain, 13–14
   panic attacks, 14
   sleep, 14
canabidiol contraindications, 115
   antibiotics, 122–123
   antidepressants and anti-anxiety medicines, 123
   blood thinners, 123
   CBD–herb–drug interactions, 121–122
   chemotherapy, 123
   ibuprofen, 124
   topical CBD, 124

canabidiol delivery methods, 115
   cannabis oil, 120–121
   capsules, 117
   inhalation, 115–117
   microemulsions, 116
   nebulisers, 116
   oral ingestion, 117–118
   skin patches, 119, 121
   sublingual, 118
   topical application, 118–120
   vaporizing, 115
canabidiol–herb–drug interactions, 121–122. *See also* canabidiol contraindications
canabidiol in practice, 159
   anxiety and post cancer malaise, 164–165
   chronic regional pain syndrome, 166–168
   fibromyalgia and cancer, 160–164
   polypharmacy and pain, 168
   severe mental health concerns, 165–166
cancer, 88
   anxiety and malaise, 164–165
   cannabis and, 103–104
   fibromyalgia and, 160–164
Cancer Act of 1939, The, 103–104
cannabichromene (CBC), 31–33
cannabidivarin (CBDV), 30–31
cannabigerol (CBG), 28–30
cannabigerovarin acid (CBGVA), 33
cannabinoid receptors, 144, 150
   type 1, 47–49
   type 2, 49–50, 95
cannabinoids, 17. *See also* canabidiol
   anandamide, 22–27
   cannabichromene, 31–33
   cannabidivarin, 30–31
   cannabigerol, 28–30
   cannabinol, 27–28
   endocannabinoids, 18
   tetrahydracannabinol, 18–20
   tetrahydrocannabivarin, 33–34
cannabinol (CBN), 27–28
cannabinolic acid (CBNA), 28
cannabis (*Cannabis sativa*), 2, 65. *See also* canabidiol; canabidiol delivery methods
   in Africa, 5
   in Ancient Egypt, 4
   Arab world, 4–5
   and ashwagandha, 97–98
   and black cohosh, 96
   and cacao, 100–101
   and cancer, 103–104
   cannabis resin, 6
   in Chinese culture, 2–3
   and echinacea, 96
   and holy basil, 95–96
   in India, 3–4
   Indian Hemp Drugs Commission, 7–9
   and lavender, 94
   legal restrictions, 10
   Marijuana Tax Act, 10
   oil, 120–121
   Persians, 4
   and rosemary, 94–95
   resin, 6
   and turmeric, 99–100
   vilification of cannabis, 7–9
cannabis extract supplements, 153
   for athletes, 153–154
   benefits offered to athlete, 155
   coronavirus, 155–157
   long COVID, 157–158
Cannabis sativa. *See* cannabis

cannaflavins, 85–87. *See also* flavonoids
capsules, 117. *See also* canabidiol delivery methods
carene, 81–82. *See also* plant secondary metabolites
caryophyllene, 67. *See also* plant secondary metabolites
catechins, 87. *See also* flavonoids
CBC. *See* cannabichromene
CBDV. *See* cannabidivarin
CBG. *See* cannabigerol
CBGVA. *See* cannabigerovarin acid
CBN. *See* cannabinol
CBNA. *See* cannabinolic acid
cell death, 26
chemotherapy, 123. *See also* canabidiol contraindications
chemovar, 60
   hybrid, 62–63
   indica subtype, 61–62
   sativa subtype, 62
chronic obstructive pulmonary disorder (COPD), 71, 138–140. *See also* health conditions and CBD
chronic regional pain syndrome, 166–168
Cimicifuga racemosa. *See* black cohosh
cocoa bean, 100
collagen connective tissue disorders, 136–138. *See also* health conditions and CBD
complementary practitioners, xv
COPD. *See* chronic obstructive pulmonary disorder
C-reactive protein, 53

crossbreeding. *See* hybridisation
Curcuma longa. *See* turmeric
CYP450. *See* cytochrome P450
cytochrome P450 (CYP450), 53–54
   subfamilies, 54

depression, 130–133. *See also* health conditions and CBD
dopamine, 24
dysmenorrhoea, 142

echinacea, 96. *See also* herbal synergy
Ehlers-Danlos syndromes, 136
endocannabinoids, 17, 35–36, 47, 51–53, 125. *See also* anandamide
   balancing, 39–45
   biphasic effect, 43–44
   CBD and interaction with, 42–43
   deficiency, 11
   dietary response, 40–41
   drugs and alcohol, 41
   endogenous ligands, 52
   failure, 38
   genetic predisposition, 41
   Herxheimer reaction, 44–45
   phytocannabinoids, 36, 42
   priming, 126
   receptors, 52
   restoring balance, 41–42
   retrograde transmission, 23
   runner's high, 42
   stress response, 39–40
endogenous ligands, 52
entourage effect, 91–92. *See also* flavonoids
Epidiolex, 31

INDEX

epilepsy, 140. *See also* health conditions and CBD
essential fatty acids, 3

FAAH. *See* fatty acid amide hydrolase
fatty acid amide hydrolase (FAAH), 23, 27, 146
fibromyalgia, 141–142. *See also* health conditions and CBD
    and cancer, 160–164
fight or flight response, 131. *See also* health conditions and CBD
flavanols, 86. *See also* flavonoids
flavanones, 86. *See also* flavonoids
flavans, 86. *See also* flavonoids
flavonoids, 85
    anthocyanidins, 86
    anthoxanthins, 85
    apigenin, 90
    aromadendrin, 87
    butin, 87
    and cancer, 88–90
    and cannabis, 90–91
    cannaflavin A, 87
    cannaflavin B and cannaflavin C, 87
    cannaflavins, 86
    catechins, 87
    entourage effect, 91–92
    flavanols, 86
    flavanones, 86
    flavans, 86
    galangin, 87
    health benefits of, 87–88
    hesperetin, 87
    isovitexin, 87
    luteolin, 88, 91
    naringin, 88
    orientin, 88
    quercetin, 88
    taxifolin, 88
    vitexin, 88

galangin, 87. *See also* flavonoids
gastrointestinal. *See also* health conditions and CBD
    conditions, 144–145
    diseases, 49
geraniol, 84. *See also* plant secondary metabolites

happy hormone, 100
health conditions and CBD, 125–128
    ADD or ADHD, 129–130
    anxiety, 130–133
    arthritis, 133
    Behçet's disease, 135–136
    collagen connective tissue disorders, 136–138
    COPD, 138–140
    depression, 130–133
    epilepsy, 140
    fibromyalgia, 141–142
    fight or flight response, 131
    gastrointestinal conditions, 144–145
    menopause, 145–147
    migraines, 147–148
    multiple sclerosis, 148–149
    pain relief, 128–129
    PCOS, 142–143
    piriformis syndrome, 152
    PMDD/PMS, 143–144
    polymyalgia rheumatic, 141–142
    priming endocannabinoid system, 126
    rheumatoid arthritis, 133–135

sciatica, 152
skin conditions, 150
sleep, 150
spinal cord injury, 150–152
stress, 130–133
hEDS. *See* hypermobile EDS
hemp, 1. *See also* canabidiol
hempseed oil, 12
herbal synergy, 93
   ashwagandha and CBD, 98–99
   cannabis and ashwagandha, 97–98
   cannabis and black cohosh, 96
   cannabis and cacao, 100–101
   cannabis and echinacea, 96
   cannabis and holy basil, 95–96
   cannabis and lavender, 94
   cannabis and rosemary, 94–95
   cannabis and turmeric, 99–100
herb–drug interactions, 55–56. *See also* metabolism
Herxheimer reaction, 44–45. *See also* endocannabinoids
Herxing. *See* Herxheimer reaction
hesperetin, 87. *See also* flavonoids
holy basil (*Ocimum sanctum*), 95–96. *See also* herbal synergy
homeostasis, 17–18, 125
HPA axis (hypothalamus–pituitary–adrenal axis), 98
humulene, 77–78. *See also* plant secondary metabolites
hybridisation, 62–63
hypermobile EDS (hEDS), 137
hypothalamus–pituitary–adrenal axis. *See* HPA axis

Ibn Sina (Avicenna), 4
ibuprofen, 124. *See also* canabidiol contraindications
Indian ginseng. *See* ashwagandha
Indian Hemp Drugs Commission, 7–9
indica, 57
   anticipated effects of, 60
   hybrid chemovars, 62–63
   indica chemovar subtype, 61–62
inene, 75–77. *See also* plant secondary metabolites
inhalation, 115–117. *See also* canabidiol delivery methods
irritable bowel, 144–145. *See also* health conditions and CBD
isovitexin, 87. *See also* flavonoids

Jarisch–Herxheimer reaction. *See* Herxheimer reaction

kidney poisoning, 75

Lamiaceae. *See* mint family
Lavandula spp. *See* lavender
lavender (*Lavandula* spp), 94. *See also* herbal synergy
limonene, 67, 72–73. *See also* plant secondary metabolites
linalool, 70–72. *See also* plant secondary metabolites
long COVID, 157–158
luteolin, 88, 91. *See also* flavonoids

Marijuana Tax Act, 10
Mechoulam, Raphael, 35
medical marijuana (cannabis), xiii
menopause, 145–147. *See also* health conditions and CBD
mental health concerns, 165–166

metabolism, 51
    and CYP450 interaction, 53
    endocannabinoid system and homeostasis, 51–53
    herb–drug interactions, 55–56
    THC metabolisation, 55
microemulsions, 116. *See also* canabidiol delivery methods
microglia cells, 50
migraines, 147–148. *See also* health conditions and CBD
mint family (Lamiaceae), 94
molluscoid pseudo tumours, 137
Moreau, J.-J., 6
multiple sclerosis, 148–149. *See also* health conditions and CBD
myrcene, 69–70. *See also* plant secondary metabolites

N-acylethanolamines (NAEs), 96
NAE. *See* N-linoleoylethanolamine
NAEs. *See* N-acylethanolamines
N-arachidonoylethanolamine (AEA), 36. *See also* anandamide
naringin, 88. *See also* flavonoids
National Institute for Health and Care Excellence (NICE), 157
nebulisers, 116. *See also* canabidiol delivery methods
neurodegenerative disorders, 53
neurotransmitters, 100–101
NICE. *See* National Institute for Health and Care Excellence
N-linoleoylethanolamine (NAE), 101
N-oleolethanolamine (OEA), 101

non-steroidal anti-inflammatory drugs (NSAIDs), 122
NSAIDs. *See* non-steroidal anti-inflammatory drugs

Ocimum sanctum. *See* holy basil
OEA. *See* N-oleolethanolamine
oral ingestion, 117–118. *See also* canabidiol delivery methods
orientin, 88. *See also* flavonoids
O'Shaughnessy, W., 5–6
osteoporosis, 145

pain relief, 128–129. *See also* health conditions and CBD
PCOS. *See* polycystic ovarian syndrome
perimenopause, 145
peroxisome proliferator-activated receptor agonist (PPARy), 157
PG/VG. *See* propylene glycol/ vegetable glycerine
phellandrene, 80–81. *See also* plant secondary metabolites
phytocannabinoids, 36, 42. *See also* endocannabinoids
phytochemicals, 17, 65. *See also* plant secondary metabolites
pinene, 67. *See also* plant secondary metabolites
piriformis syndrome, 152. *See also* health conditions and CBD
plant-derived pharmaceutical anticancer agents, 89
plant secondary metabolites, 65
    camphene, 79–80
    carene, 81–82

caryophyllene, 67, 73–75
geraniol, 84
humulene, 77–78
limonene, 67, 72–73
linalool, 70–72
myrcene, 69–70
phellandrene, 80–81
pinene, 67, 75–77
pulegone, 82–83
sabinene, 83–84
terpenes, 66–68
terpineol, 82
terpinolene, 78–79
plant terpenoids, 65. *See also* plant secondary metabolites
PMDD. *See* premenstrual dysphoric disorder
PMS. *See* premenstrual dysphoric disorder
polycystic ovarian disease. *See* polycystic ovarian syndrome
polycystic ovarian syndrome (PCOS), 142–143. *See also* health conditions and CBD
polymyalgia rheumatic, 141–142. *See also* health conditions and CBD
polypharmacy, 56
and pain, 168
post-traumatic stress disorder (PTSD), 97
PPARy. *See* peroxisome proliferator-activated receptor agonist
PPIs. *See* proton pump inhibitors
premenstrual dysphoric disorder (PMDD), 143–144. *See also* health conditions and CBD

propylene glycol/vegetable glycerine (PG/VG), 115
proton pump inhibitors (PPIs), 122
PTSD. *See* post-traumatic stress disorder
pulegone, 82–83. *See also* plant secondary metabolites

quercetin, 88. *See also* flavonoids

RCGP. *See* Royal College of GPs
retrograde transmission, 23–24. *See also* anandamide
rheumatoid arthritis, 133–135. *See also* health conditions and CBD
Ritalin, 39
rosemary (*Rosmarinus off.*), 94–95. *See also* herbal synergy
Rosmarinus off. See rosemary
Royal College of GPs (RCGP), 157
runner's high, 24–25, 42. *See also* anandamide

sabinene, 83–84. *See also* plant secondary metabolites
salbutamol, 116
sativa, 57
    anticipated effects of, 60
    chemovar subtype, 62
    hybrid chemovars, 62–63
sciatica, 152. *See also* health conditions and CBD
Scottish Intercollegiate Guidelines Network (SIGN), 157
SIGN. *See* Scottish Intercollegiate Guidelines Network
skin. *See also* canabidiol delivery methods; health conditions and CBD

conditions, 150
hyperextensibility, 137
patches, 119, 121
sleep, 150. *See also* health conditions and CBD
spinal cord injury, 150–152. *See also* health conditions and CBD
stress, 130–133. *See also* health conditions and CBD
sublingual, 118. *See also* canabidiol delivery methods

taxifolin, 88. *See also* flavonoids
terpenes (volatile oils), 65–66, 159. *See also* plant secondary metabolites
terpineol, 82
terpinolene, 78–79
tetrahydracannabinol (THC), 3, 10–11, 18, 28, 33, 55
metabolisation, 55
therapeutic value, 19–20
tetrahydrocannabivarin (THCV), 33–34
tetrahydrocannabivarin carboxylic acid (THCVA), 33
THC. *See* tetrahydrocannabinol
THCV. *See* tetrahydrocannabivarin
THCVA. *See* tetrahydrocannabivarin carboxylic acid

Theobroma cacao, 100
topical application, 118–120. *See also* canabidiol delivery methods
topical CBD, 124. *See also* canabidiol contraindications
tramadol, 128
TRPV-1 receptors, 26
tulsi. *See* holy basil
turmeric (*Curcuma longa*), 99–100. *See also* herbal synergy

ulcerative colitis, 144–145. *See also* health conditions and CBD

vanilloid receptors. *See* TRPV-1 receptors
vaporizing, 115. *See also* canabidiol delivery methods
vitexin, 88. *See also* flavonoids
volatile oils. *See* terpenes

Withania somnifera. *See* ashwagandha

zingiberene, 99

Printed by Printforce, United Kingdom